THE COMPLETE GUIDE TO

SUSPENDED FITNESS TRAINING

3. **Door anchors**: While all suspension straps will come with some sort of anchoring solution as part of the basic equipment package, not all straps come with a door-anchoring solution. A door anchor is usually a short length of webbing with a block or cylinder of hard plastic at one end. The webbing attaches to the anchoring carabiner and the plastic block is used to sit over the top of a solid, secure door which is then closed. The closed door now serves as a useful, indoor-anchoring solution. This provides a workout solution for use in the home, hotel, office or other scenario. Although a door anchor is not essential, it does provide a useful function for individuals looking to use suspended fitness training as a portable training solution.

4. **Pulley systems**: Another more advanced option available within the suspended fitness market is the inclusion of a pulley as the central feature. This feature essentially is a single-anchor-suspension system, but instead of a loop that the main strap passes through, a pulley is used instead. This usually means that one-inch-wide webbing is not the main component of the system, instead, it is normally a type of rope that attaches the handles and runs through the central pulley. The inclusion of a central pulley means that the handles can be used to control the length of rope on either side of the pulley as the rope is drawn back and forward through the pulley itself. This significantly increases the degree of instability and increases the amount of effort and strength required to control and balance the system while in use. A suspended-pulley system is less suitable for beginners, but as skill and strength increase, a pulley system does provide a more challenging option.

BENEFITS OF SUSPENDED FITNESS TRAINING

Performing exercises from a suspended rope or strap places the body under physical stress as the muscles try to resist the pull of gravity and control the desired movements and exercises. When consistently applied as part of a structured exercise programme suspended fitness training can elicit numerous physical benefits. An overview of the potential training benefits associated with suspended training are as follows:

- Increased muscular strength and endurance
- Improved muscle tone and activation
- Improved movement coordination
- Improved lean body mass
- Increased flexibility
- Improved functional range of motion
- Improved capacity for muscle force generation without injury
- Improved communication between nerves and muscles

Performing physical exercise while suspended from straps or ropes creates a training environment unlike any other kind of exercise. One of the key physiological differences this creates is an increase in the number of muscles that need to be active to control movement at the primary joints involved in an exercise. This is known as co-contraction. Co-contraction can be observed when muscles on both sides of a joint or group of joints contract to help increase joint rigidity and to prevent unwanted movement. Most people likely remember their first time venturing on to an ice rink and their efforts to reduce the level of instability by stiffening up the body and reducing the range of movement at the joints to help maintain balance and prevent a fall. This is a classic example of co-contraction. Increased levels of co-contraction are commonly created within the fitness environment through the use of unstable fitness equipment, such as stability balls, BOSU, air disks or wobble boards. In most cases, these tools are used for increasing muscle activation around the mid-section of the body during exercise and as a result the exercises feel harder than when performed on solid, stable ground. Often this simple increase in muscular workload is used as a justification for how effective the unstable equipment is for training and may convince some people that they are a better mode of training. However, just like walking on ice leads to a stiffer, reduced range of movement when walking or skating for the first time, the use of unstable training mediums, including suspended fitness training, not only increases muscle activation but tends to reduce and limit range of motion in an effort to remain stable. It is important that the use of suspended training is applied correctly so that joint range of motion is not adaptively decreased, leading to reduced function and poor joint health.

Stability balls, BOSU and wobble boards all require the user to be on top of the equipment by means of standing, sitting or lying during exercise and thereby creating a stimulus from the feet, hips or back passing up through the body. The nervous system has to respond by controlling the instability at the feet or hips first and then progressively up through the body as one joint movement affects the one above it. In contrast, suspended fitness training provides a slightly different stimulus and requires the user to hang underneath the training equipment from unstable straps or ropes. Being suspended from the arms with the feet still in contact with the floor means that the instability is occurring above the body with the nervous system needing to control movement at the hands down through each successive joint. Therefore, in most exercises, suspended fitness training creates a top-down nervous-system response rather than a ground-up response. These are subtle differences, but nonetheless help create important changes in exercise stimulus that the body needs to adapt to.

In many suspended exercises the body is controlled between two primary contact points: the feet in contact with the ground and the hands gripping the handles of the equipment. Gravity is constantly acting upon the rest of the body, and muscle contraction occurs to hold the knees, hips and back in good alignment during performance. This is the reason fans of the equipment consider suspension exercises to provide excellent core training as the muscles that surround the hips, torso and back are often involved in the performance of correct exercise technique. While numerous suspended fitness exercises will train the core muscles by default, there are also many specific exercises that are able to target the trunk muscles more intensely, which certainly justifies the claim that suspension equipment provides an excellent means of training the core muscles.

As a result of increased levels of co-contraction around the limbs, multi-directional movement, coordination of multiple body parts and greater involvement of the core muscles, suspended fitness training offers a refreshing and meaningful form of total body workout.

EXERCISE SAFETY

As with many forms of exercise, there are a number of safety risks associated with suspended fitness training. Many of these risks, when managed appropriately, can be substantially reduced, ensuring that exercise within a suspended environment can continue with minimal concern for harm or injury.

Perhaps one of the more common safety risks that often concern a new user is that the suspension equipment will break or fail causing a fall and potential injury. While this is indeed a possibility, the build quality of most modern suspension equipment is sufficient that the risk of strap or hardware failure is very low. As discussed earlier, the breaking point of a standard one-inch-wide polypropylene strap is still a reassuring 400kg (880lbs) with nylon and polyester straps being much stronger. It is unlikely that this high level of stress will be placed through a suspension kit during normal physical exercise. In most cases the strength of the handles, carabiners and connecting links can often take several hundred kilograms and are unlikely to fail either. This may not provide a 100 per cent guarantee that suspension equipment will never break, although the risk of a strap failing will increase if the equipment becomes damaged or worn. If the strap is allowed to rub against another surface or object during use then this can begin to wear the material, create small pulls in the fabric and weaken the strap at the site of damage. The more the material becomes damaged, the lower the level of force it will take to exceed the breaking point. The same can be said for the handles or connecting links. Therefore, it would be considered good practice to visually check the suspended equipment before each use to ensure there are no obvious defects that may increase the risk of it breaking and causing potential injury to the user.

Perhaps a more likely safety risk is that an individual's own physical ability fails them and they fall and become injured. Some examples of this could include:

- Loss of grip on the handles during an exercise that leads to an undesirable forwards or backwards fall
- Loss of balance during a single-leg exercise and a joint becomes sprained or a muscle strained
- Poor spinal alignment during an exercise places higher stress on the spinal discs and increases the risk of injury to the back

While each of these examples identifies a realistic safety concern, all can be managed effectively with some simple guidance. Ensuring that an exercise is selected to match an individual's current ability can help to minimise risk considerably. Starting with the easier exercises, and gradually progressing to more difficult exercises as technique and ability improves, is a sensible rule to follow in any form of exercise. Injury during exercise is much more common when an individual tries to engage in an exercise that is several steps ahead of their current ability. As fitness, strength and technical ability improve with practice and gradual progress, the risk of injury when performing more complex exercises reduces due to an individual's greater ability.

One last area of risk that can be managed with relative ease concerns setting the equipment up for use. First and foremost is the selection of a suitable anchoring point. In a typical gym setting, suspension equipment is usually anchored to a purpose-built frame or it is attached to anchoring points that are securely fixed to the wall. These will likely have been tested to provide sufficient strength to support the maximal forces that could be placed through a suspension system. Using suspended fitness equipment at home, in an office or outdoors in a public park will require the selection of an appropriate anchor point. It is vital that the selected anchor point can easily support the user's body weight and that it is firm and rigid. It is also important that a selected anchor point will allow sufficient space for the performance of exercise without the risk of collision with any other object or person. The anchor point must be high enough overhead to allow for correct performance of exercise. The required height can vary a little across the different types of equipment, but in most cases a suitably strong anchoring point around two metres high works well. When training inside in a non-gym environment a door often provides a very useful anchor point. It is important that the door is strong enough itself combined with a solid, sturdy door frame. In most cases it is probably best not to anchor suspension equipment over hollow plywood or very lightweight doors. Solid doors with strong frames are most desirable. It is also important that once the equipment is anchored over a door that the direction of pull will close the door rather than pull it open.

HEALTH AND SAFETY CONSIDERATIONS

Prior to beginning an exercise regime it is important to screen oneself for any risk to participation. Most fitness clubs require their clients to complete a PAR-Q (Physical Activity Readiness Questionnaire) form which will highlight any fundamental contraindications to exercise and indicate whether an individual should be referred to a doctor before engaging in exercise. If exercising from home it would be wise to honestly review your own health to ensure you are in a good position to start a training programme. Seek help from a medical practitioner if you are unsure about any specific health markers.

The following steps offer a sensible quick checklist to run through before participation in suspended fitness training:

- check the strength of the object that the straps will be anchored to. This MUST be able to withstand the user's total body weight and any other pulling or tugging forces created during exercise
- check the suspension equipment for any signs of wear and tear, including the webbing, carabiners and handles
- ensure the selected exercise environment provides a flat, non-slip and stable surface with plenty of room to train
- once the straps are anchored into position test they can withstand the load thoroughly before commencing exercise
- ensure hands are dry and non-greasy to reduce the risk of losing grip. Wearing training gloves may also help with increasing grip if needed
- wear appropriate training shoes that provide sufficient grip on the floor or training surface
- select a flat, dry, non-greasy, non-dusty training surface to provide suitable grip for the feet during each exercise
- technique is of fundamental importance when performing suspended exercises. Only progress to more advanced exercises once technique and ability have been mastered
- while strength and stability training is suitable for the majority of people, some population groups should be more careful and may need to avoid this form of training, including:
  - stage 2 and 3 hypertensive clients
  - arthritic and osteoporotic clients
  - pregnant women
  - obese, sedentary clients

SUSPENDED ANGLES

3

At first glance it may not appear that hanging from a polyester strap and performing a few rows is particularly scientific, but the reality is a whole field of scientific study is devoted to human movement, forces and angles. This area of science is known as biomechanics. When considered from a scientific perspective, suspended fitness training involves many different biomechanical elements such as angular forces, gravitational pull, pivot points, momentum, the pendulum effect, lever length and the effects of ground reaction. A brain-bending study of human biomechanics is not for everyone, but gaining a rudimentary knowledge of some of the basic principles will certainly help in providing an appreciation of how different suspended exercises can affect and influence the user.

There are four primary biomechanical concepts that will affect the load and degree of difficulty an individual may experience when performing suspended fitness exercises. These four elements are:

• body height and mass
• angle of loading
• leverage and mechanical advantage
• the pendulum effect

BODY HEIGHT AND MASS

In many cases, suspended fitness training involves hanging from straps while the feet remain fixed against the floor serving as a fulcrum or pivot point. An individual's height affects the distance between the two primary pivot points: the feet fixed on the ground, and the handles attached to the end of the straps, which is the point where force is applied. The longer the distance between these two points, the greater the amount of effort that needs to be applied to overcome the same body weight. This is because the length from the ground-based pivot point to application of force at the handles, known as the moment arm, impacts upon the degree of torque. Torque is simply the amount of turning force that is generated around a pivot point.

Using a wrench to turn a bolt provides a classic example of the principle of torque at work. The amount of twisting force required to loosen a bolt is set at a fixed threshold regardless of whether a short- or long-handled wrench is used. A long-handled wrench (moment arm) helps to amplify the torque needed to loosen the bolt and makes it feel easier than using a short-handled wrench. Selecting the long-handled wrench allows the user to benefit from the longer moment arm, making

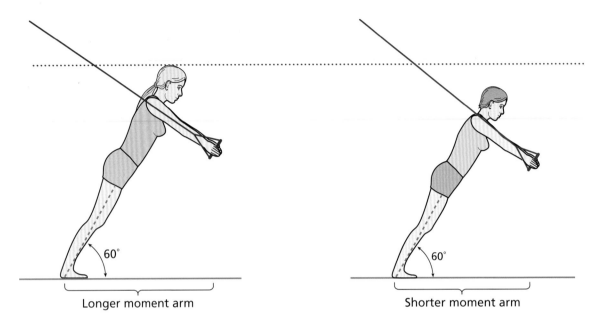

60°

Longer moment arm

60°

Shorter moment arm

Figure 3.1 Effect of height on moment arm and load

the force of application feel easier to turn the bolt, but this is traded for a larger distance that the force will need to be applied for each revolution of the bolt. A short-handled wrench would feel harder to turn, but the measured circumference of one complete turn of a small wrench would be much less than a single circular turn of a long-handled wrench. The apparent decrease in application of force when using the long wrench is exchanged for an increase in distance covered to loosen the bolt. Therefore, the force required using a long-handled wrench may be lower, but it needs to be applied for a greater period of time and the work performed is in reality the same.

There is a difference when applying this to a human being working with suspension straps. During an exercise the muscular force that needs to be generated must overcome the individual's

own body weight in respect to the torque or turning force created by gravitational pull. This is a little different to the resistance of a tight bolt needing to be loosened by a wrench. Gravity is creating the torque, while the individual needs to resist this turning force. A shorter individual will have a lower degree of torque to resist, whereas a taller individual will need to resist a higher amplification of torque, which will likely feel harder for the same relative angle of load. A taller individual also has longer arms, which decreases mechanical advantage and makes the force of production a bit more difficult for the same relative load.

Imagine two individuals who are both 80 kilograms in weight, but one is 10 inches taller. They have set up the suspension straps from the same overhead anchor point with their feet positioned so as to be at the same body angle of 60 degrees.

The taller individual would in fact need to put in greater effort to overcome the larger level of torque that is amplified by the gravitational pull due to their height.

In respect to body mass, it is important to consider some of the typical gender differences and where each carries the proportion of their weight. Men tend to carry more of their total mass in the upper body with broader shoulders and narrower hips compared to women. This means a man has to overcome an increased amount of torque compared to a woman of the same body weight and height, due to a greater proportion of their body mass being positioned further away from the pivot point. However, with greater muscle mass in the upper body a man should also be able to cope with this increased torque sufficiently in comparison to women, who tend to have less upper body mass and less upper body strength.

ANGLE OF LOADING

Suspended fitness training exercises can be performed across a wide range of different angles. Many exercises even require movement that changes the angle during each repetition. The angle of the body or attached body part between the ground and the straps will affect the intensity of the exercise and the total workload experienced. If the centre of gravity during a rowing or pressing exercise is located closer to the feet, then a larger percentage of total body weight will be loaded through the legs. The closer that centre of gravity moves towards the hands, the larger the percentage of total body weight passed through the upper limbs. Therefore, in most cases the following general rule seems to apply: the closer to vertical during exercise the greater the load through the lower extremities, whereas the closer to horizontal during exercise the greater the load through the upper extremities.

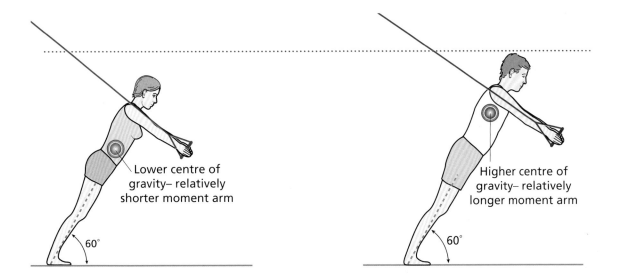

Figure 3.2 Effect of centre of gravity on moment arm

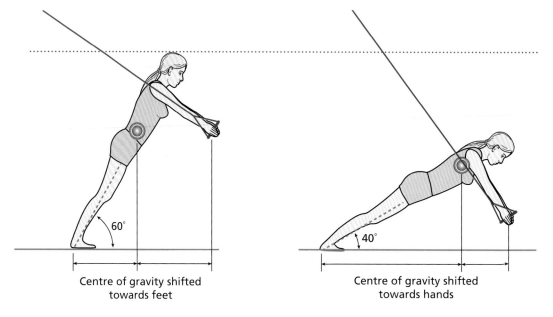

Centre of gravity shifted
towards feet

Centre of gravity shifted
towards hands

Figure 3.3 Effect of loading angle on centre of gravity

LEVERAGE AND MECHANICAL ADVANTAGE

A basic appreciation of the three types of levers and how they can change exercise intensity will help in understanding the forces that a client will experience when performing different types of suspended exercises. The three lever types are named simply by the position of the load in relation to the point where effort is applied and the position of the pivot.

First-class leverage is not a common feature of suspended training, considering that most of these kinds of exercises involve holding the handles with feet fixed on the floor while requiring gravity and body weight to provide resistance. Second and third-class leverage are a more common part of suspended fitness training.

It's useful to understand the difference between second and third-class leverage. Second-class lever exercises are set up so that the lever system

	Position 1	Position 2	Position 3	Mechanical example
1st Class	Load	Pivot	Effort applied	Seesaw
2nd Class	Pivot	Load	Effort applied	Wheel barrow
3rd Class	Pivot	Effort applied	Load	Tongs

Figure 3.4 caption to come

magnifies the effort that is required and makes the exercise feel more difficult. Third-class lever exercises are set up so that the lever system enhances the velocity of movement and the effort required to perform the exercise may feel easier.

When the resistance arm and the effort arm are identical in length then the lever merely transfers the effort and speed of movement exactly as it is applied but in a different direction. This is exactly what happens to make the playground seesaw work. A shorter resistance arm and longer effort arm provides a mechanical advantage that makes the effort experienced by the user much lighter, but the force created at the opposite end of the lever is greatly magnified. Using a screwdriver to open a tightly closed container, like a paint pot lid, works on this principle of magnifying force generation as described above. When the resistance arm is longer than the effort arm this creates

a mechanical advantage that magnifies the velocity of movement, but in so doing makes the load experienced by the user feel heavier. Think about a fisherman trying to reel in a large fish using a fishing rod. The fisherman will hold the handle near the bottom of the rod (short-effort arm) and will need to work harder to hold the rod firm against a pulling fish. However, the long length of rod beyond the gripping point (long-resistance arm) is necessary as it allows the fish to be pulled in rapidly when it tires and stops pulling against the line. This method and design provides a mechanical benefit to more easily land a big fish.

The following diagram brings this back to fitness and exercise by showing examples of basic pressing and pulling exercises and how the leverage varies. The second-class exercise places the body between the pivot and the pushing point, increasing the load, whereas the third-class

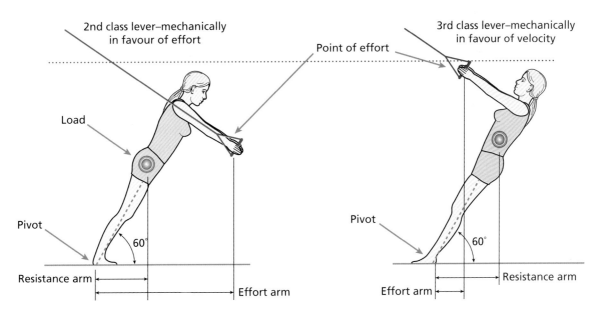

Figure 3.5 Types of lever utilised during suspended fitness training

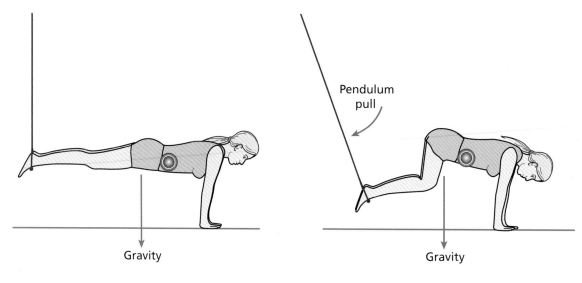

Figure 3.6 The pendulum effect

exercise has the pulling point between the body and the pivot point at the feet, reducing load and making greater velocity of movement possible. This can help explain why even when an individual is angled at 60 degrees for either a suspended push or pull exercise the intensity of the exercise can vary significantly, with the pushing exercise often feeling harder for the same body angle.

THE PENDULUM EFFECT

A pendulum is a weight that is suspended from a pivot point so that it can swing freely after it has been pushed to one side, and gravity influences the load. As a pendulum is brought into motion it swings outward and upward in an equidistant arc from the pivot. The weight at the end of the rope or lever is subject to the restoring forces of gravity that constantly pull it downward in an effort to draw it back to the original perpendicular position. Once the load is pulled off centre it is

subject to a degree of momentum that swings the load as a result of the gravitational forces acting upon it.

Certain suspended fitness exercises are affected by pendulum-like motion and the effects of gravity can be amplified to increase intensity and load. An example of an exercise that exploits the pendulum effect is the suspended plank and other related variations. If the plank is performed with the feet held in the straps directly under the pivot point then the only workload that the body has to resist against is the gravitational pull on the hips as the individual attempts to keep the body in good alignment. However, by inching the position of the body forwards so that the feet are now 12 to 18 inches in front of the pivot or anchor point while holding the plank position the body has two forces to resist: the downward pull of gravity at the hips as well as the pendulum pull of gravity against the feet in the straps. This additional force makes the same exercise feel increasingly more difficult.

SUSPENDED MOBILITY

4

Immediately before starting to exercise, it is important to warm up in order to increase muscular warmth, pliability and tissue activation. This will help to reduce early exercise injury risk and improve muscular performance. A short aerobic warm-up, like cycling on a stationary bike or jogging on a treadmill, should be included to achieve increased blood flow, greater oxygen delivery and improved muscle temperature. However, these activities do not sufficiently elongate muscle tissue and stimulate muscle-cell activation at the extreme end-ranges of joint motion. Therefore, it is vital to ensure that the muscles to be used in a workout are introduced to end-of-range, reduced-load movement exercises during the warm-up. Holding static stretches as part of the warm-up is largely ineffective at preparing the body for exercise so will not be advised as part of the warm-up/mobility component of a suspended fitness workout.

Using dynamic mobility gradually to build up the range of movement at each of the joints in the body is vital. The selected dynamic movements should gradually move the joints closer to end-range and ease the muscle tissue into a lengthened, activated state. Each dynamic movement should start slowly within a comfortable range and gradually increase to a moderate pace while simultaneously increasing the range of motion. This will help to slowly encourage an increase in muscle length and mobilise the joint while still maintaining muscle warmth, heart rate and the other beneficial effects of the aerobic warm-up.

Suspended fitness equipment can be used for muscle and joint mobilisation. It can provide support in order to help reduce the load passing through the muscles as well as helping to maintain balance and position during mobility exercises. The intention is to select the dynamic mobilisations that are most appropriate to the exercise session that is to follow. Trying to carry out the entire set of mobilisation movements included in this chapter would take too much time and limit the main workout. If the exercise focus for a single workout is squats and pushing movements then it makes sense to select dynamic mobilisations that target the muscles involved in these movements, such as the quadriceps, gluteals, hamstrings, calf complex and pectorals. Programme design will be discussed in more depth in Chapter 9.

The following series of mobility exercises will help to provide an effective library of movements to warm up the major muscles and groups of muscles that are likely to be needed in a typical fitness regime.

Body part: Lower leg

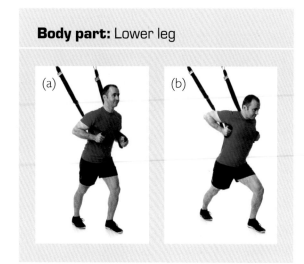

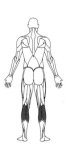

Muscles
Calf complex

Set-up
Straps anchored high and set to an equally short length. Standard handles attached

Positioning
Place straps under both armpits with handles gripped immediately either side of the chest

Technique
- Facing away from the anchor point, lean forward against the straps with the feet in a long split stance
- Drive the front knee forward while keeping the back heel on the ground to lengthen the back leg calf muscle tissue
- Return to the start position
- Perform 10–15 reps then repeat on the other leg

Body part: Back of thigh

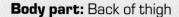

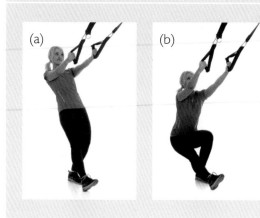

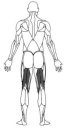

Muscles
Hamstrings

Set-up
Straps anchored high and set at equally short length. Standard handles attached

Positioning
Face towards the anchor point holding the handles at arm's length and lean back to place the straps under tension

Technique
- With one leg supporting your body weight hold the other leg straight in front of the body with the knee very slightly unlocked and foot in contact with the ground
- Lower the body downwards, bending at the hips until a stretch is felt on the back of the straight leg, lengthening the hamstrings
- Rise up and lower again to move into the stretch for each repetition
- Perform 10–15 reps then repeat on the other leg

Body part: Inner thigh

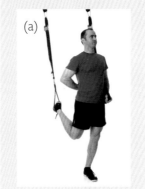

(a)　(b)

Body part: Front of thigh

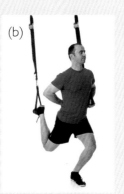

(a)　(b)

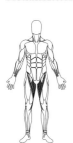

Muscles
Hip adductors

Set-up
Straps anchored high and set at equally short length. Standard handles attached

Positioning
Face towards the anchor point holding the handles at arm's length and lean back to place the straps under tension

Technique
- With one leg supporting your body weight hold the other leg straight out to the side of the body with foot in contact with the ground
- Lower the body downwards until a stretch is felt on the inside thigh of the straight leg, lengthening the hip adductors
- Rise up and lower again to move into the stretch for each repetition
- Perform 10–15 reps then repeat on the other leg

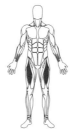

Muscles
Quadriceps

Set-up
Straps anchored high and one set short and the other set at a medium length. Short strap with a handle, medium strap with foot loop attached/used

Positioning
Stand facing away from the anchor point with left foot placed in the foot loop behind the body with the knee bent and the other strap held in the right hand

Technique
- Use the higher strap to maintain balance
- Bend the standing right leg to lower the body downwards, keeping the left hip pushed forward to feel a stretch through the front of the thigh
- Rise up and lower again to move into the stretch for each repetition
- Perform 10–15 reps then repeat on the other leg

19

Body part: Front of hips

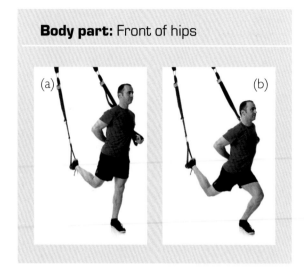

(a) (b)

Body part: Outer hip

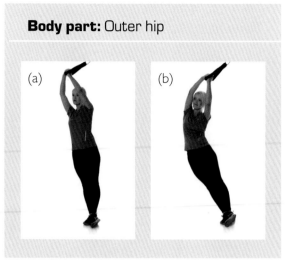

(a) (b)

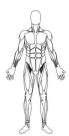

Muscles
Iliopsoas

Set-up
A single strap is anchored high and set at full length. Foot loop attached

Positioning
Begin in a split kneeling lunge position with the foot of the back leg placed in the attached foot loop

Technique
• Keeping the forward foot rooted to the ground drive the knee into a deep lunge position
• Drive the hips forward while reaching overhead and behind to feel a stretch across the front of the back leg hip
• Drive back and forward again to move into the stretch for each repetition
• Perform 10–15 reps then repeat on the other side

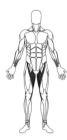

Muscles
Hip abductors

Set-up
Single strap anchored high and set at a short length. Standard handle attached

Positioning
Begin standing sideways in relation to the straps with right foot crossed over the left and holding the handle with both hands overhead creating tension in the strap

Technique
• Maintaining the overhead hold on the handle allow the right hip to move outwards away from the straps until a stretch is felt across the outer right hip
• Draw hips back inwards and repeat
• Perform 10–15 reps then repeat on the other side

Body part: Buttocks

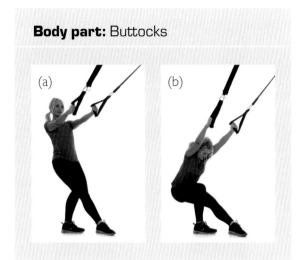

(a) (b)

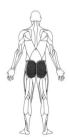

Muscles
Gluteus Maximus

Set-up
Straps anchored high and set at an equal medium length. Standard handles attached

Positioning
Begin by standing in a long split stance facing the anchor point and gripping both handles, one in each hand

Technique
- Shift the front foot across to the inside of the body about 6 inches (15cm) past the centre of the body
- Lean back and with extended arms support the body while lowering into a deep lunge position
- Simultaneously look down at the ground and allow the upper body to face downwards while driving the hips down and backwards
- Rise back up and repeat for each repetition
- Perform 10–15 reps then repeat on the other side

Body part: Buttocks

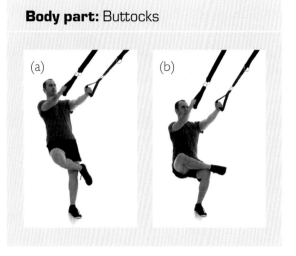

(a) (b)

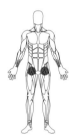

Muscles
Piriformis and deep hip rotators

Set-up
Straps anchored high and set at equally short length. Standard handles attached

Positioning
Begin standing on one leg facing towards the anchor point gripping both handles, one in each hand

Technique
- Raise the non-supporting leg up and cross it over the knee with the outer ankle resting on the knee of the stance leg and the other leg allowed to drop outwards to the side
- Holding the crossed leg position, lower the stance leg downwards into a single-leg squat position supporting body weight with the straps
- Lower until a stretch is felt deep on the outer hip of the crossed leg
- Perform 10–15 reps then repeat on the other side

Body part: Lower and mid back	**Body part:** Mid and upper back

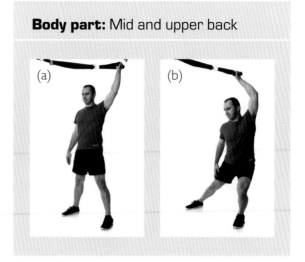

(a) (b) (a) (b)

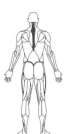

Muscles
Erector spinae

Set-up
Straps anchored high and set at equally short length. Standard handles attached

Positioning
Stand with feet together facing the anchor point and gripping both handles, one in each hand

Technique
- Keeping both feet firmly fixed on the ground bend at the hips while keeping the knees straight
- Allow the hips to drop down and backwards while supporting the body with the straps and a high overhead grip
- Allow the spine and back to elongate and be held in traction while tucking the chin into the chest
- Draw hips forwards and return to the start position then repeat
- Perform 10–15 reps

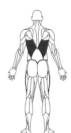

Muscles
Latissimus dorsi

Set-up
Straps anchored high and set at equally short length. Standard handles attached

Positioning
Stand sideways in relation to the straps with a wide stance and hold one of the handles overhead in the hand furthest away from the straps

Technique
- Shift body weight over to one side and descend into a side lunge on the leg furthest away from the straps
- Simultaneously side bend, allowing the overhead arm to be drawn across to the other side, stretching out the target muscle
- Return to the start position and repeat
- Perform 10–15 reps then repeat on the opposite side arm

Body part: Abdominals

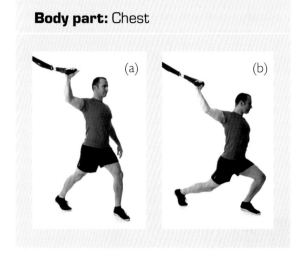

(a)　(b)

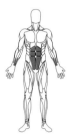

Muscles
Rectus abdominis

Set-up
Straps anchored high and set at equally short length. Standard handles attached

Positioning
Begin in a split stance facing away from the straps with both hands holding one of the handles overhead

Technique
- Inch forward until the strap is under tension
- Lower the body downwards and forwards into a lunge, allowing the arms to be drawn back and up stretching out the abdominals
- Rise up again releasing the arms slightly and repeat
- Perform 10–15 reps then repeat on the other side

Body part: Chest

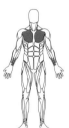

Muscles
Pectoralis major

Set-up
Straps anchored high and set at equally short length. Standard handles attached

Positioning
Begin facing away from the anchor point holding one handle out to the side and above the head, then inch forward so the straps are under tension

Technique
- Step forward with one leg and drop into a lunge
- Allow the arm to be drawn back, stretching the pectorals on that side
- Drive back up out of the lunge and repeat, but step lunge on the opposite leg
- Perform 10–15 reps

Body part: Upper arm

Body part: Shoulders

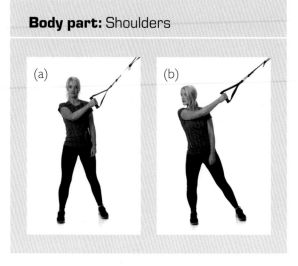

(a) (b)

(a) (b)

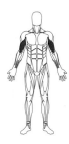

Muscles
Biceps brachii

Set-up
Straps anchored high and set at equally short length. Standard handles attached

Positioning
Stand in a split stance facing away from the anchor point and holding one strap directly behind the lower back

Technique
• Step forward and drop down into a lunge, allowing the arm to rise up behind the body keeping the chest lifted throughout
• Keep the arm narrow and close to the midline of the body and the elbows locked
• Lower down until a stretch is felt through the biceps
• Rise back to the start and repeat alternating the lunge leg
• Perform 10–15 reps then repeat on the other side

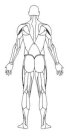

Muscles
Posterior deltoids

Set-up
Straps anchored high and set at equally short length. Standard handles attached

Positioning
Stand sideways in relation to the straps and hold one handle across and in front of the body at shoulder height

Technique
• Step laterally away from the strap pulling it tight and stretching the posterior deltoid
• Step back and then repeat
• Perform 10–15 reps then repeat on the other side

SUSPENDED EXERCISE BASICS

5

The exercises contained within this chapter provide a foundation to suspended fitness training. If suspended training is a new part of your exercise regime it would be wise to begin with these starter exercises and master the basics before progressing to the next chapter where more advanced exercise progressions will be covered. At this early stage it is important to pay close attention to the technique of each exercise to achieve the correct execution before moving on to the more advanced exercises. Mastering the basic exercise techniques explained in this chapter will pay dividends when encountering the next level of exercise progressions, therefore focusing on these early exercises and spending time on them will be well worth it. The exercises chosen to help lay this foundation will be categorised using basic human movement patterns, which are also linked to the most common types of suspended movement training exercises. The human movement patterns are simply:

- pushing
- pulling
- squatting
- lunging
- core control

The movements available at the core of the body include flexion, extension, lateral flexion and rotation of the spine, which will all be referred to as core control. Many of the exercises will also involve movement across three directions or planes – the sagittal, frontal and transverse planes. It is helpful to learn these three terms as they help explain movement within the exercise technique sections.

- Sagittal – movement directed anterior and posterior, or forwards and backwards
- Frontal – movement directed medial and lateral, or side to side both in and out
- Transverse – movement directed through horizontal rotation in either direction

Combining human movement patterns with different planes of motion helps to address important functional aspects of exercise. This not only creates an interesting exercise library from which to draw upon, but also ensures that the exercises relate to common human movements that will improve daily function as well as develop strength and fitness.

Each exercise has a 'Quick guide' simply detailing how to perform the exercise correctly, followed

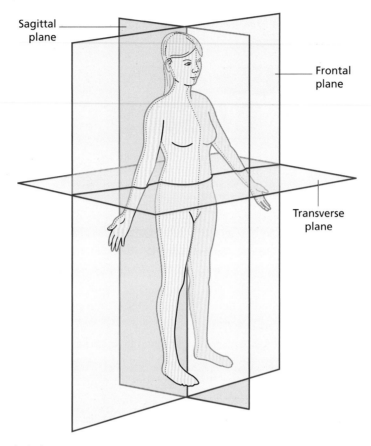

Figure 5.1 Anatomical planes

by a more in-depth 'Technical tips' section that will provide a higher level detail to master and understand. Feel free to choose – keep it simple with the 'Quick guide' or jump in deep and geek out with the 'Technical tips.' The exercise technique chapters focus primarily on learning how to perform the various exercises. Chapter 9 will explain and offer guidance on how to draw upon the exercise library to build an effective physical training programme and offers several examples of exercise programming for different ability levels and objectives.

EQUIPMENT SET-UP

It is important to invest a little time to ensure that the suspension kit is set up correctly before use. Get into the habit of checking the straps thoroughly during set-up to ensure there is no damage to the equipment. Looking for frayed straps, smalls pulls in the material, bent or broken carabiners and cracks in the handles should become a habit each time the equipment is pulled out of the bag and is being prepared for use. Minor damage that does not immediately weaken the strength of the straps should be monitored over time to ensure that it does not progress to the point where it may compromise the overall strength of the system. More significant damage to straps or attachments may require repair, a replacement part or in the worst-case scenario perhaps the system needs to be completely replaced. When using suspended fitness straps safety should always be the first priority.

During set-up it is always worth taking a few extra seconds to check the anchoring carabiners are closed securely, the straps are anchored correctly and not twisted and that the handles are connected and secure. As previously discussed, some suspension systems have two straps that need to be anchored separately, while other systems may only require a single-anchor point. There are different ways in which the straps can be anchored to an object. The first involves wrapping the anchor strap several times around a secure object and clipping both looped ends into the anchoring carabiners. The second involves wrapping the anchor strap once around the object, feeding one end of the anchor strap through the loop at the other end and then attaching the free end of the anchor strap to the anchoring carabiner. Both methods of anchoring a system are acceptable and it may come down to preference as to which you prefer.

It is good practice once set-up is complete to double check the buckle adjustment is secure so the straps don't slip during use, all the carabiners are completely locked shut so as not to catch and fray the straps and finally that the straps have been firmly pulled and tugged to ensure they are fixed in place and will not suddenly slip or become loose during use. Developing these good habits when setting up suspension equipment will help to provide a level of safety and care that will increase exercise safety and also the longevity of the suspended fitness straps themselves.

EXERCISE CHALLENGE RATINGS

Each exercise contained within the basic and advanced exercise chapters has an exercise 'Challenge rating' to help provide guidance on how easy or difficult an exercise is to perform. The exercise 'Challenge rating' will be determined by a combination of two other scores, the 'Technique rating' and the 'Intensity rating'. The intensity and technique scores will be rated out of four with a rating of one being considered easy or low and a rating of four considered as very difficult or high. The 'Challenge rating' will be calculated by simply adding the technique and intensity ratings together to provide a range of one to eight as an overall score for each exercise. These scores will help to select the appropriate exercises when designing a suspended fitness training programme that will match an individual's current ability or competency levels.

PUSH EXERCISES

Exercise 1 Chest press

(a)   (b)

Target muscles: Pectorals
and triceps
Technique rating: 1
Intensity rating: 1
Challenge rating: 2

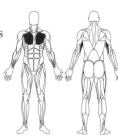

Set-up

Straps anchored high and set at equal length on each strap from mid to short. Standard handles attached

Positioning

Feet in a neutral position and fixed behind the body slightly in front of the anchor point. Face away from the anchor point and grip the handles with arms in front of the body at shoulder height

Quick guide

- Lean forward into the straps so that the arms take the load
- Bend at the elbows and shoulders, bringing the body forward until the chest is almost in line with handles
- Push back against the handles, driving the body back to the start position and repeat
- Keep the chest lifted up and other key joints in good alignment

Technical tips

- The sharper the angle that is created between the user and the ground, the greater the load that will be experienced through the muscles (pectorals, triceps and deltoids)
- Ensure that as the elbows and shoulders bend into the downward portion of the press that they remain directly behind the hands to help keep the wrists straight and ensure better joint alignment position
- Good joint and spinal alignment must be maintained throughout the press with ankles, knees, hips and spine all holding fixed to allow the body to form an effective lever that pivots on the ball of the foot during the pressing movement
- Avoid the hips dropping forward with gravity as this will place undue pressure on the lower back and increase injury risk

Exercise 2 Chest flye

(a)   (b)

Target muscles: Pectorals and deltoids
Technique rating: 1
Intensity rating: 2
Challenge rating: 3

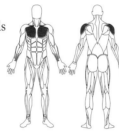

Set-up
Straps anchored high and set at equal length on each strap from mid to short. Standard handles attached

Positioning
Feet placed in neutral stance and fixed behind the body slightly anterior to the anchor point. Grip handles with the arms straight and in front of the body at shoulder height

Quick guide
- Lean forward into the straps so that the arms support the weight of the body
- Open the arms outwards in a wide lateral arc, controlling their posterior motion until the hands are out to the side and almost level with the body
- Drive the arms forward in front of the chest bringing the hands back in front of the body until they meet again in the middle
- Keep the chest lifted up and other key joints in good alignment

Technical tips
- The sharper the angle that is created between the user and the ground the greater the load that will be experienced through the muscles (pectorals and anterior deltoids)
- Ensure that as the shoulders move during both the outward and inward arc of the flye motion that the wrist, elbow and shoulder joints are maintained in strict alignment, the elbow joint being kept slightly soft so it does not lock out
- Good joint and spinal alignment must be maintained throughout the press with ankles, knees, hips and spine all holding fixed to allow the body to form an effective lever that pivots on the ball of the foot during the flye movement
- Avoid the hips dropping forward with gravity as this will place undue pressure on the lower back and increase injury risk
- Avoid the shoulders drifting upward into an externally rotated position with the hands finishing above the elbows towards the end of the outward arc. This creates a difficult and less stable position for the shoulders that can increase injury risk

Exercise 3 Suspended press-up

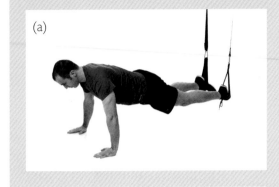

(a)

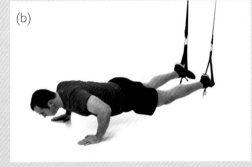

(b)

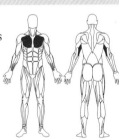

Target muscles: Pectorals and triceps
Technique rating: 1
Intensity rating: 2
Challenge rating: 3

Set-up

Straps anchored high and set at equal length to the long position. Foot loops attached

Positioning

Standard press-up position with hands flat on the ground, feet suspended laces down in the foot loops and the feet directly underneath the anchor point

Quick guide

- Bend at the elbow and shoulders, controlling the descent against gravity to lower the body down until the elbows are out to the sides at right angles, then drive upwards back to the top position with the elbows locked out
- Hold the body in good alignment from feet to shoulders throughout the press-ups

Technical tips

- This exercise will require the user to already have the ability to perform a full press-up as normal with feet on the ground. Suspending the feet in the loops will increase the load and difficulty of the exercise compared to normal press-ups by shifting a greater portion of body weight on to the arms and by decreasing the stability of the body overall
- Avoid the hips dropping downward with gravity as this will place undue pressure on the lower back and increase injury risk. Keep the ankles, knees, hips and shoulders in alignment parallel with the ground throughout each press-up
- Avoid rapidly descending or collapsing into the downward motion of the press-up. Strive to control the downward part of the movement and transition smoothly into the upward movement

Exercise 4 Suspended triceps dip

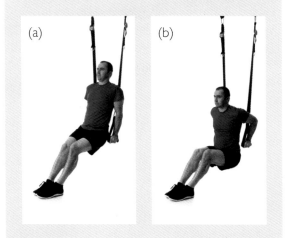

(a) (b)

Target muscles: Deltoids and triceps
Technique rating: 2
Intensity rating: 2
Challenge rating: 4

Set-up

Straps anchored high and set at equal length from mid to long position. Standard handles attached

Positioning

Stand between the straps and squat down to then grip the handles and hold them tight in beside each hip. Keeping the arms straight down at the sides allow body weight to pass through the arms and walk the feet out in front of the body until the legs are straight out in front of the body with the heels in contact with the ground.

Quick guide

- Lower the body downward by bending at the elbows and shoulders until the elbows are at right angles behind the body
- Drive back upward locking the elbows out at the top of each repetition
- Keep the chest lifted throughout the exercise
- Ensure the legs and lower body remain relaxed with heels in contact with the ground

Technical tips

- It is important to move the arms in pure shoulder extension keeping the elbows tight against the body. If the elbows drift out wide then the downward motion causes the shoulders to move into abduction instead of extension and more of the load will be taken by the pectorals, reducing the work done by the triceps
- The legs should be relaxed and knees extended, pivoting on the heels during each repetition. For the full effect the legs should not be supporting any body weight
- If it is too difficult to perform a full-suspended dip then the soles of the feet can be placed against the floor and the knees bent slightly to allow a small portion of the weight of the body to be supported by the legs, reducing the workload on the triceps and making the exercise manageable

Exercise 5 Overhead triceps press

(a)

(b)

Target muscles: Triceps
Technique rating: 2
Intensity rating: 1
Challenge rating: 3

Set-up

Straps anchored high and set at equal length from mid to long position. Standard handles attached

Positioning

Begin by standing facing away from the anchor point, holding the handles with both arms directly overhead. Lean forward so that both straps are under tension.

Quick guide

- Keep the upper arms from shoulder to elbow fixed in a vertical position and maintain alignment from feet to shoulders throughout the exercise
- Bend at the elbows so the body drops forward under control until the elbows are at right angles and hands are behind the head still holding handles firmly
- Press against the handles and straighten the arms back until they are directly overhead again and the body has been pulled back up to the original start position

Technical tips

- It is important that the shoulders remain fully flexed and the upper arms are kept in a vertical position tight to the sides of the head. If the elbows drift out wide during the downward motion of the body then more of the load will be taken by the pectorals and latissimus dorsi which will reduce the work done by the triceps
- Sagging at the hips and extending through the lower back must be avoided as good alignment is essential. If the load and intensity experienced by the triceps is too great then extending the lower back lengthens the abdominals stimulating a contraction which can aid the positive movement back to the start position. This can be avoided by ensuring the feet are fixed at an appropriate distance from the anchor point so that angle of loading of the body is suitable to match the strength of the triceps without the need to cheat or use bad technique

PULL EXERCISES

Exercise 6 Narrow grip hanging row

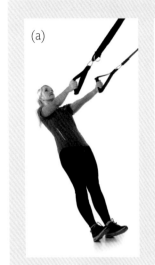
(a)

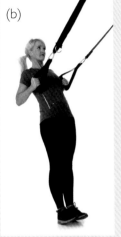
(b)

Target muscles:
Latissimus dorsi
and biceps
Technique rating: 1
Intensity rating: 1
Challenge rating: 2

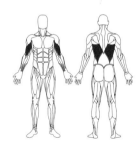

Set-up
Straps anchored high and set at equal length from short- to mid-range. Standard handles attached

Positioning
Feet are fixed slightly in front of the anchor point while facing towards the straps. Grip handles at arm's length

Quick guide
- Lean back to place the straps under tension
- Pull against the straps driving the chest towards the anchor point
- Draw the elbows back keeping them close to the sides of the body
- Keep body alignment from feet to shoulders throughout the exercise

Technical tips
- Pure shoulder extension must be emphasised during the row to ensure the greatest load is created by the large latissimus dorsi muscle. Allowing the shoulders to lift up towards the ears or the elbows to drift wide will incorrectly shift some of the workload to the trapezius and surrounding muscles and reduce the work done by the latissimus dorsi.
- While elbow flexion is a part of the movement it should always be secondary to shoulder extension, too much emphasis on elbow flexion will draw the handles in towards the shoulder joint and work the biceps very hard. The handles should be drawn in towards the lower ribcage so that shoulder extension is the focus and the latissimus dorsi takes up the majority of the work.
- Avoid the hips dropping downward with gravity as this will increase the likelihood of rowing high towards the shoulders and over-stressing the biceps.
- Keep the ankles, knees, hips and shoulders in alignment throughout each row pivoting either at the ankle joint or rocking on the heel

Exercise 7 Single grip narrow row and reach

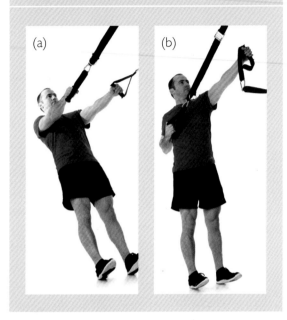

(a) (b)

Target muscles:
Latissimus dorsi and biceps
Technique rating: 2
Intensity rating: 2
Challenge rating: 4

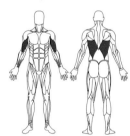

Set-up
Straps anchored high and set at equal length from short- to mid-range. Standard handles attached

Positioning
Both feet are fixed to the ground in a wide position slightly in front of the anchor point while facing towards the straps. Grip the handles at arm's length.

Quick guide
- Lean back bringing the straps under tension
- Pull against the handle with the lead arm, lifting the body up and drawing the elbow strongly behind the body while the free arm is quickly drawn forwards and reaches up towards the anchor point
- Allow the body to naturally rotate while reaching up with the free arm
- Control the descent back to the start position
- Keep good alignment through spine and other joints of the body

Technical tips
- Shoulder extension must be emphasised during the row to ensure the greatest load is created by the large latissimus dorsi muscle. Drawing the elbow and arm back towards the lower ribs and hip, rather than pulling the hand towards the shoulder, will help to achieve this
- The upward pulling motion needs to be performed powerfully in order to generate enough motion to reach the free arm high towards the anchor point, however the descent must be controlled and gravitational pull resisted
- Avoid the hips dropping downward with gravity as this will allow the shoulder to move into flexion and increase the risk of rowing high towards the shoulder joint and over-stressing the biceps
- Keep the ankles, knees, hips and shoulders in alignment throughout each row pivoting either at the ankle joint or rocking on the heel

Exercise 8 Wide hanging row

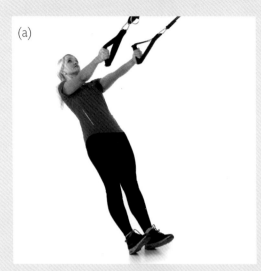

(a)

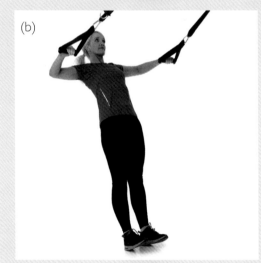

(b)

Target muscles: Trapezius, deltoids and biceps
Technique rating: 2
Intensity rating: 1
Challenge rating: 3

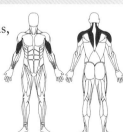

Set-up

Straps anchored high and set at equal length from short- to mid-range. Standard handles attached

Positioning

Feet are fixed slightly in front of the anchor point while facing towards the straps. Grip handles at arm's length

Quick guide

- Lean back and place the straps under tension
- Pull against the straps driving the chest towards the anchor point
- Draw the elbows back and wide keeping them high and level with the shoulders
- Keep body alignment from feet to shoulders throughout the exercise

Technical tips

- The emphasis of this exercise is to move the shoulders and draw back the upper arms through horizontal extension and to retract the scapula
- Elbows must remain high and aligned at shoulder level, but care must be taken not to destabilise the shoulder joint by lifting the shoulders up towards the ears
- Avoid the hips dropping downward with gravity as this will increase the likelihood of rowing high towards the shoulders and over-stressing the biceps
- Keep the ankles, knees, hips and shoulders in alignment throughout each row, pivoting either at the ankle joint or rocking on the heel

Exercise 9 Reverse flye

(a)

(b)

Target muscles: Trapezius and deltoids

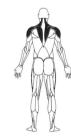

Technique rating: 1
Intensity rating: 2
Challenge rating: 3

Set-up

Straps anchored high and set at equal length from short- to mid-range. Standard handles attached

Positioning

Feet grounded in a neutral position slightly in front of the anchor point and face towards the straps. Grip handles at arm's length

Quick guide

- Lean back and place the straps under tension
- Maintain relatively straight arms at the elbow and pull the body upwards by drawing the arms wide and back at shoulder level while driving the chest forwards, the arms and body forming a 'T' shape
- Control the descent back to the start
- Keep good alignment through spine and other joints of the body

Technical tips

- It is easy to be tempted to use other joint motion to swing and initiate the primary movement at the shoulders. This needs to be avoided and kept to a minimum. If the load is too great to draw back into horizontal extension at the shoulders without swinging first then inch the feet further back away from the anchor point to reduce the load that has to be overcome when performing the flye movement
- The elbows do not need to be locked out into full extension during this exercise, but can be kept slightly soft just shy of lock out so as to reduce the sheer forces passing through the joint
- Avoid the hips dropping downward with gravity as this will allow the shoulders to move into flexion and lead to an undesirable hip swing motion to help initiate horizontal extension
- Keep the ankles, knees, hips and shoulders in alignment throughout each flye pivoting either at the ankle joint or rocking on the heel

Exercise 10 Hanging biceps curl

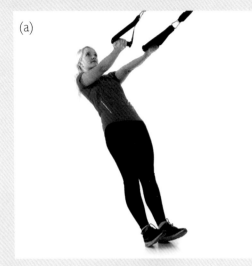

(a)

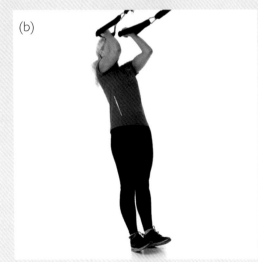

(b)

Target muscles: Biceps
Technique rating: 1
Intensity rating: 1
Challenge rating: 2

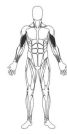

Set-up
Straps anchored high and set at equal length on each strap from mid to long. Standard handles attached

Positioning
Stand facing the anchor point gripping both handles at arm's length leaning back to place tension through the straps

Quick guide
- Keep the upper arms fixed in front at right angles to the body and maintain alignment of the body from feet to shoulders
- Bend the elbows and draw the hands to the sides of the forehead pulling the body upwards towards the anchor point
- Straighten the arms and lower the body under control back to the original start position

Technical tips
- It is important that the only movement that draws the body up is elbow flexion. If the angle of loading is too great that the biceps cannot complete the movement alone then it is likely the compensatory movement to help lift the body upwards will be pulling the shoulders through into extension similar to a narrow row. The correct angle of loading to match bicep capacity must be selected
- Maintaining good body alignment and avoiding the hips sagging backwards is also important. Bending the hips even a small amount when the arms are outstretched will likely lead to a compensatory hip drive to lift the body and reduce the load felt by the biceps during their pulling action. This may be another sign that the angle of loading is too great for the biceps to cope with and should be adjusted to match biceps capacity.

Exercise 11 Single arm biceps curl

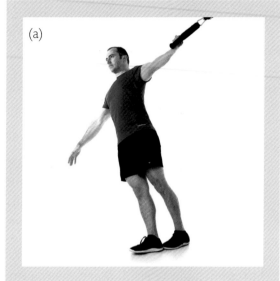

(a)

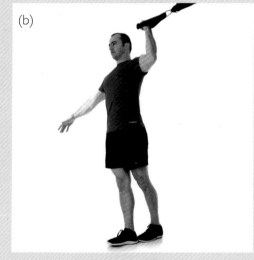

(b)

Target muscles: Biceps
Technique rating: 2
Intensity rating: 1
Challenge rating: 3

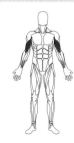

Set-up
Straps anchored high and set at equal length on each strap from mid to long. Standard handles attached

Positioning
Stand in a small split stance turned 90 degrees away from the anchor point gripping a single handle at arm's length out to the side of the body while leaning sideways to place tension through the strap

Quick guide
- Keep the upper arm fixed out to the side at a right angle to the body and maintain alignment of the body from feet to shoulders
- Bend the elbow and draw the hand in towards to the side of the head pulling the body upwards towards the anchor point
- Straighten the arms and lower the body under control back to the original start position

Technical tips
- It is important that the only movement that draws the body up is elbow flexion. As this is a single arm exercise if the angle of loading is too great the biceps of the working arm will not be able to complete the movement. The correct angle of loading to match biceps capacity must be selected. Excess load will likely lead to poor form to compensate
- Maintaining good body alignment and avoiding the hips sagging sideways is important to ensure that other muscles around the hips are not contracting to help generate momentum and ease the bicep load

SQUAT EXERCISES

Exercise 12 Suspended squat

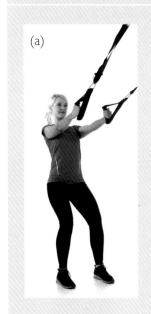
(a)

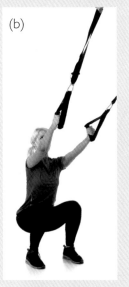
(b)

Target muscles:
  Quadriceps and gluteals
Technique rating: 1
Intensity rating: 1
Challenge rating: 2

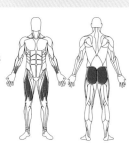

Set-up
Straps anchored high and set at equal length from short- to mid-range. Standard handles attached

Positioning
Begin with feet fixed in a neutral position approximately 18–24 inches (45–60 cm) in front of the anchor point. Face towards the anchor point and grip the handles at arm's length.

Quick guide
- Lean back and place the straps under tension
- Bend at the hips and lower the body downwards while simultaneously bending at the knees until a squat position is reached with knees and hips at right angles
- Keep the arms at full length and lean back against the straps throughout the squat movement so that they can support balance and body weight to the degree required
- Drive the body upwards with the legs and return back to the start position
- Keep the chest lifted and shoulders drawn back throughout the movement

Technical tips
- The focus of the suspended squat is to help individuals learn to master squat mechanics so that they can squat in perfect form without any exercise aids in future
- Good squat technique is a matter of optimally balancing downward body movement and the effects of gravity. Observe the change of angle at the tibia and the spine – these body parts should always be parallel throughout the downward and upward movements of a squat. This maintains centre of gravity over the feet and ensures good balance
- Feet should be maintained at normal hip width apart when squatting. A wide stance is often used to allow greater squat depth, but this is only a compensation of poor range of motion, particularly lack of forward ankle motion. Where ankle range is lacking this should be properly addressed with flexibility work
- Keep knees tracking in line with the first and second toes throughout each squat

Exercise 13 Overhead squat

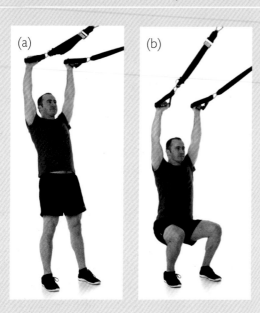

Target muscles:
   Quadriceps, gluteals
   and deltoids
Technique rating: 2
Intensity rating: 1
Challenge rating: 3

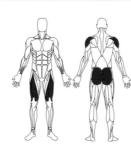

Set-up

Straps anchored high and set at equal length from short- to mid-range. Standard handles attached

Positioning

Begin with feet fixed in a neutral position approximately 18–24 inches (45–60 cm) in front of the anchor point. Face towards the anchor point and grip the handles directly overhead at arm's length.

Quick guide

- Lean back, so that the high arms are supporting body weight while maintaining good spinal alignment
- Bend at the hips and lower the body downwards while simultaneously bending at the knees until a squat position is reached with knees and hips at right angles
- Keep the arms at full length above the head and lean back gently against the straps throughout the squat movement to provide balance and challenge posture
- Drive the body upwards with the legs and return back to the start position
- Keep the chest lifted and shoulders drawn down and back throughout the movement

Technical tips

- The purpose of the overhead squat is to provide a postural challenge using a relatively simple exercise technique and to load the body gently in this position
- The tibia angle should be fairly parallel with the back and overhead arm angle throughout the downward and upward movements of a squat. This will help provide balance and challenge posture
- Feet should be maintained at normal hip width apart and knees tracking in line with the first and second toes throughout each squat

Exercise 14 Single-leg squat

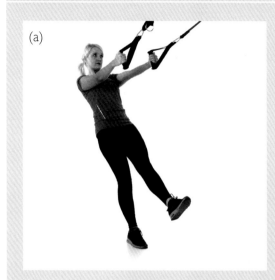

(a)

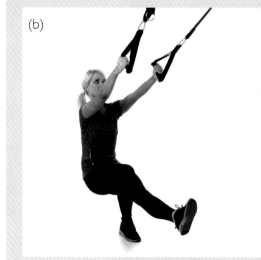

(b)

Target muscles:
Quadriceps and gluteals
Technique rating: 2
Intensity rating: 2
Challenge rating: 4

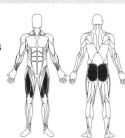

Set-up
Straps anchored high and set at short- to mid-range. Standard handles attached

Positioning
Begin facing towards the anchor point in a standing single-leg balance position with the non-standing leg held slightly in front of the body. The handles are held at arm's length, leaning back slightly with the straps under tension

Quick guide
- Bend the hip and knee of the stance leg to lower the body down into a deep single-leg squat, seeking to bend the knee beyond a right angle
- The non-weight-bearing leg is held off the ground out in front of the body during the squat
- Drive back upwards to the starting single-leg standing position and repeat
- Keep good spinal alignment while holding the handles at arm's length and maintaining tension in the straps throughout

Technical tips
- The single-leg squat lends well to getting into an effective deep squat position as the support of the straps allows both balance and additional help when driving up back out of the squat position
- Ensure the chest is kept lifted and spinal alignment is maintained during the squat. While a deep squat position is desirable it should not come at the expense of a loss of back position, especially if the pelvis rolls posteriorly and drags lower back out of alignment
- The stance leg knee should track over the first and second toes throughout the squat movement

Exercise 15 Suspended squat jump

(a)

(b)

(c)

Target muscles:
Quadriceps, gluteals and
calf complex

Technique rating: 1
Intensity rating: 3
Challenge rating: 4

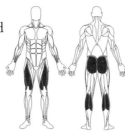

Set-up

Straps anchored high and set at equal length from
short- to mid-range. Standard handles attached

Positioning

Begin with feet fixed in a neutral position approximately 18–24 inches (45–60 cm) in front of the
anchor point. Face towards the anchor point and
grip the handles at arm's length.

Quick guide

- Lean back and place the straps under tension
  while maintaining good body and spinal
  alignment
- Bend at the hips and quickly lower the body
  downwards while simultaneously bending at
  the knees until a squat position is reached with
  knees and hips close to right angles
- Keep the arms at full length, gripping the
  handles and lean back against the straps
  throughout the squat jump movement so that
  they can provide balance
- Drive the legs powerfully upwards and slightly
  back, moving into the air, landing again softly
  on the balls of the feet to then return back to
  the start position
- Keep the chest lifted and shoulders drawn back
  throughout the movement

Technical tips

- Increasing speed of movement and adding
  ground reaction forces to an exercise tends to
  highlight weaknesses in form and technique
  that may not yet be mastered but are less obvious when the exercise is performed at slower
  speeds and exercise intensities. Extra attention
  to good form is needed during squat jumps
- Avoid excessive bending at the hips in the
  downward loading phase of the movement
  where the angle of the spine exceeds the angle
  of the tibia at the lowest point of the movement.
  This loading pattern tends to create anterior
  momentum when exploding into the jump.
  Seek to keep tibia and spinal angles parallel as
  much as possible when loading the jump
- Feet should be maintained at normal hip width
  apart when loading into a squat jump and when
  landing so as to be prepared to go straight into
  the next repetition
- Keep knees tracking over the first and second
  toes throughout each squat jump and aim to
  land on the ground with the balls of feet and
  soft knees that bend and absorb the forces of
  impact

Exercise 16 Squat jump start

(a)

(b)

(c)

Target muscles:
Quadriceps and calf complex
Technique rating: 2
Intensity rating: 3
Challenge rating: 5

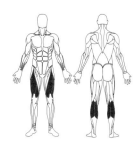

Set-up
Straps anchored high and set at equal length from short- to mid-range. Standard handles attached

Positioning
Begin with feet fixed in a neutral position slightly in front of the anchor point. Face away from the anchor point, pass the straps under the armpits and grip the handles close to the body on either side of the chest.

Quick guide
- Lean forwards allowing the straps to support body weight while maintaining spinal alignment
- Bend the hips and knees quickly lowering the body downwards into a partial squat position, loading the legs ready to jump
- Drive the legs powerfully upwards, jumping into the air as though trying to leap forwards
- Move with the straps at their end-range as they arc upwards and back towards the ground
- Land on the balls of the feet and with soft knees to reduce impact and return to the start position

Technical tips
- A degree of trust in the straps is required during this exercise as they are essential to control the anterior upward drive that guides the body up in the air and then down again to regain contact with the ground
- Squat depth during the loading phase immediately before jumping does not need to be a deep as the standard squat or squat jump. The quick loading phase is closer to a half squat with relatively greater flexion coming from the knees and ankles respectively and slightly less flexion from the hips
- Feet should be hip width apart and keep the knees tracking over the first and second toes during the loading and landing phases of the exercise
- Keeping the chest lifted throughout and the body fairly rigid in the air will help to keep control of movement in the desired direction
- Avoid the legs swinging forward immediately after the jump while the body is in the air as this will throw out the landing and quick resetting for the next repetition

LUNGE EXERCISES

Exercise 17 Suspended lunge

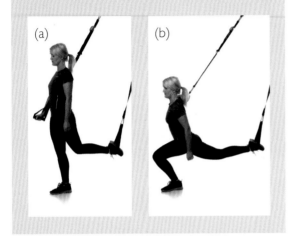

(a) (b)

Target muscles: Gluteals and quadriceps
Technique rating: 2
Intensity rating: 2
Challenge rating: 4

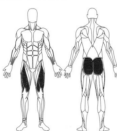

Set-up

Straps anchored high with one set at full length and the other medium. A foot loop should be attached to the long strap and a handle to the medium strap

Positioning

A single foot is fixed to the ground in a neutral position about three feet in front of and facing away from the anchor point. The other foot is placed in the foot loop attached to the strap with the sole of the foot facing upwards. The opposite hand to the foot in the loop grips the handle in front of the body to aid balance

Quick guide

- Move forward so that the rear foot in the loop pulls the strap forward a little
- Bend at the stance leg knee and hip to move the body downward, dropping into a deep lunge position
- Reach the arm holding the handle a little further in front of the body to help maintain balance and encourage a little more bend at the hip
- Drive back up to the start position

Technical tips

- Maintaining balance during this exercise may be a challenge in the early stages, especially when the muscles involved are beginning to fatigue after a number of repetitions and stabilisation at the joint becomes less controlled. Care should be taken to prevent unwanted falls and the supporting strap used for safety when needed
- It is acceptable, even desirable, to perform the suspended lunge with a greater degree of flexion at the hip than at the ankle. The forward arm reach helps to encourage a shift of centre of gravity forwards over the lead leg and it helps to increase the degree of hip flexion which in turn increases muscular contraction at the gluteals
- The knee of the lead leg should track over the first and second toes during the lunge. If the knee has a tendency to drop inwards at the bottom of the lunge it can be helpful to alter the arm reach. Performing a rotational reach over the lead leg and around to the side can help to better balance the body and reduce the inward knee drift

Exercise 18 Stabilisation lunge

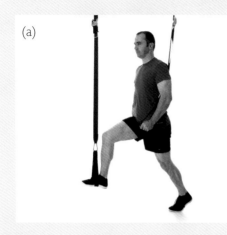

(a)

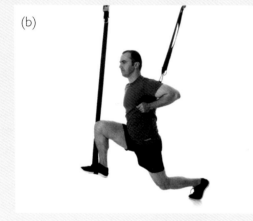

(b)

Target muscles: Gluteals
    and quadriceps
Technique rating: 2
Intensity rating: 2
Challenge rating: 4

Set-up

Straps anchored high with one set at full length the other short. A foot loop should be attached to the long strap and a handle to the medium strap.

Positioning

A single foot is fixed to the ground in a neutral position directly below the anchor point. The other foot is placed in the foot loop attached to the strap in front of the body with the sole facing downwards and toes pointing forwards. The opposite hand to the foot in the loop grips the handle close to the shoulder to aid balance

Quick guide

- Bend the knee and hip of the leg in the foot loop to move the body downward and forwards, dropping into a lunge position
- The lunging leg will be less stable in the foot loop and will require constant small corrections to keep control and stabilise each repetition
- Use the short strap to help maintain balance, but be careful not to pull the body upwards so as to reduce the effects of body weight on the lunging leg
- Drive back up to the start position under control and repeat

Technical tips

- Maintaining balance during this exercise may be a challenge in the early stages especially when the muscles involved are beginning to fatigue after a number of repetitions and stabilisation at the joint becomes less controlled. Care should be taken to prevent unwanted falls and the supporting strap used for safety when needed
- The knee off the lead leg should track over the first and second toes during the lunge

Exercise 19 Suspended side lunge

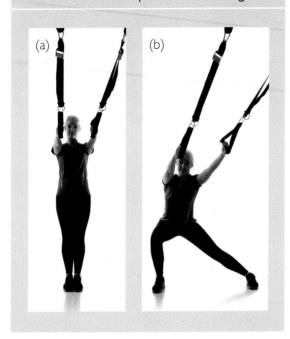

(a) (b)

Target muscles:
Quadriceps, abductors and gluteals
Technique rating: 2
Intensity rating: 1
Challenge rating: 3

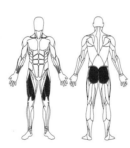

Set-up
Straps anchored high and set at mid-range. Standard handles attached

Positioning
Start in a standing, neutral stance position. The handles are held at arm's length facing towards the anchor point, leaning back with the straps under tension.

Quick guide
- Take a wide lateral step and bend the knee and hip of the lead leg to lower into a side lunge
- Drive powerfully with the lead leg upward and back inwards to return to the start position
- Keep good spinal alignment throughout and avoid pulling with the arms to help return to the middle
- Either perform all the repetitions on one leg then repeat on the opposite side or alternate sides on each repetition until a full set is complete

Technical tips
- A side or frontal lunge requires that the position of both feet remain pointed directly forwards in the start and the lunge positions. Care should be taken to ensure the feet do not externally rotate during the lunge
- As the lead leg is lowering into the lunge, the trail leg needs to remain with the sole of the foot in contact with the ground, the knee extended and locked out so that the leg remains straight and body weight is being carried primarily by the lead leg
- Flexing of the trail leg knee can often indicate that the trail leg is still partially supporting body weight. It is better to take some of the load through the straps and to perform the exercise correctly on the lead leg only than to allow the trail leg to perform poorly

CORE EXERCISES

Exercise 20 Suspended box position

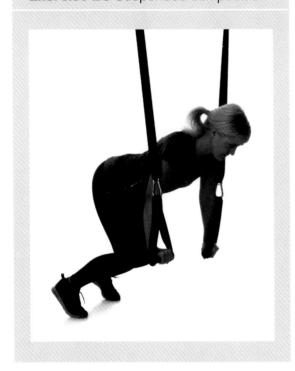

Target muscles:
Abdominals and deltoids

Technique rating: 1
Intensity rating: 2
Challenge rating: 3

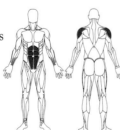

Set-up

Straps anchored high and set at long range. Handles are attached

Positioning

Begin kneeling on all fours with the head directly beneath the anchor point and hands gripping the handles

Quick guide

- Lift the knees off the ground so that the body is suspended between the hands holding the handles and the toes on the ground
- Ensure that good spinal position is maintained and the hips and knees are at 90-degree angles
- Hold this position for the desired length of time while maintaining a comfortable breathing rhythm
- Lower the knees back to the floor to bring the body to rest

Technical tips

- Keep the hips, spine and shoulders in good alignment and as stable as possible during the box position. The head should also be in line with the eyes, which are looking directly at the ground. Avoid looking up and extending the cervical vertebrae
- As the core muscles begin to fatigue the body will tend to revert to its dominant postural position where it feels strongest, which may not always be in good spinal alignment. Avoid the pelvis rolling forwards and arching the lower back. Avoid arching the spine upwards and rounding shoulders. Avoid twisting the spine as a result of one hip or knee sagging lower than the other

Exercise 21 Suspended box crawl

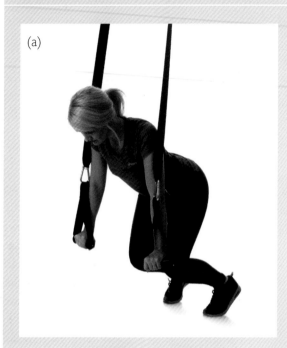
(a)

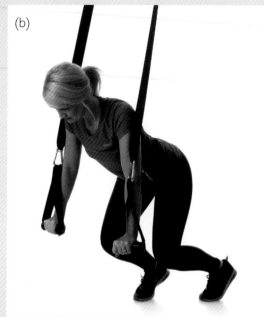
(b)

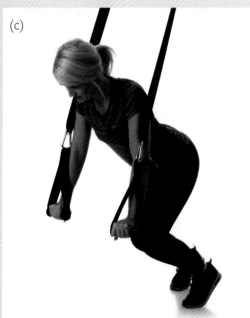
(c)

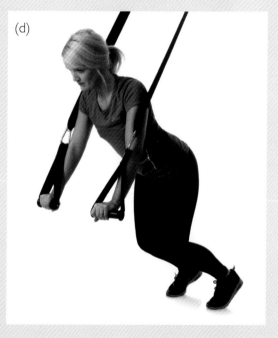
(d)

Target muscles:
Abdominals and deltoids
Technique rating: 2
Intensity rating: 2
Challenge rating: 4

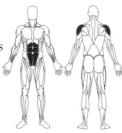

Set-up
Straps anchored high and set at long range. Handles are attached

Positioning
Begin kneeling on all fours with the head directly beneath the anchor point and hands gripping the handles

Quick guide
- Lift the knees off the ground so that the body is suspended between the hands holding the handles and the toes on the ground
- Ensure that good spinal position is maintained and the hips and knees are at 90-degree angles
- While maintaining strong and stable arm and spinal positions begin taking small 2–3 inch (5–7 cm) steps forward with the feet, crawling the body forward 18–24 inches (45–60 cm) and then inching back to the start position
- Lower the knees back to the floor to bring the body to rest

Technical tips
- Keep the hips, spine and shoulders in good alignment and as stable as possible during the box crawl. The head should also be in line with the eyes looking directly at the ground. Avoid looking up and extending the cervical vertebrae
- The steps with the feet must be small, just inching the body forward a little at a time rather than taking large strides
- The straps will begin to arc upward slightly creating a pendulum effect that the arms must control and resist in order to maintain the desired box position
- As the core muscles begin to fatigue the body will tend to revert to its dominant postural position where it feels strongest, which may not always be in good spinal alignment. Avoid the pelvis rolling forwards and arching the lower back. Avoid arching the spine upwards and rounding shoulders. Avoid twisting the spine as a result of one hip or knee sagging lower than the other

Exercise 22 Suspended plank

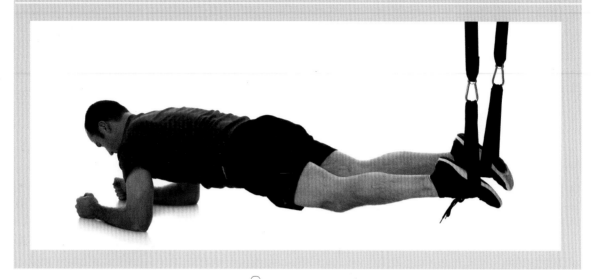

Target muscles: Abdominals and iliopsoas
Technique rating: 1
Intensity rating: 2
Challenge rating: 3

Set-up
Straps anchored high and set at long range. Foot loops attached

Positioning
Begin lying face down with feet set in the foot loops and elbows and forearms on the ground

Quick guide
- Lift the hips off the ground until they are in alignment with the shoulders and feet in the loops and there is good spinal position
- Hold this position for the desired length of time while maintaining a comfortable breathing rhythm
- Lower the hips and torso to the floor to bring the body to rest

Technical tips
- Keep the ankles, knees, hips, spine and shoulders in good alignment and as stable as possible during the plank hold. The head should also be aligned with the eyes looking directly at the ground. Avoid looking up and extending the neck
- As the core muscles begin to fatigue the body will tend to revert to its dominant postural position where it feels strongest, which may not always be in good spinal alignment. Avoid the pelvis rolling forwards and arching the lower back. Avoid arching the spine upwards and rounding shoulders. Avoid twisting the spine as a result of one hip sagging lower than the other

Exercise 23 Suspended hip bridge

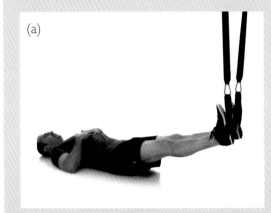

(a)

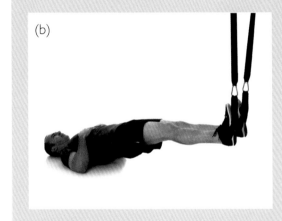

(b)

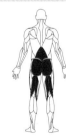

Target muscles: Gluteals, hamstrings and lumbar erectors
Technique rating: 1
Intensity rating: 2
Challenge rating: 3

Set-up
Straps anchored high and set at long range. Foot loops attached

Positioning
Begin lying face up with heels or feet set in the foot loops directly under the anchor point, legs together, knees and hips bent and arms held across the chest

Quick guide
- Lift the hips off the ground until they are in alignment between the shoulders and knees and there is good spinal position. Body position will be angled downward towards the head.
- Hold the bridge position for a 5–10 seconds then lower the hips back to the ground and repeat
- Keep the knees bent at 90 degrees throughout the exercise

Technical tips
- Keep the knees, hips, spine and shoulders in good alignment and as stable as possible during the elevated hold or hip bridge position. The head should be relaxed and in contact with the ground throughout. Avoid looking up and flexing the neck
- The first signs of fatigue will likely be that it becomes too difficult to keep the knees in a 90-degree position as the hamstrings lose strength and the knees begin to extend. The hips may also begin to drop out of alignment. As the posterior core muscles begin to fatigue the body will tend to revert to its dominant postural position where it feels strongest, which is often not optimal alignment. Avoid the pelvis rolling forwards drawing the lower back into an arched position. If form cannot be corrected then the exercise should cease

Exercise 24 Reverse plank with splits

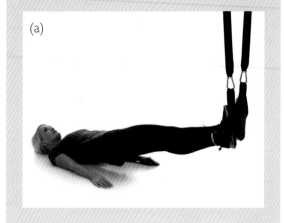

(a)

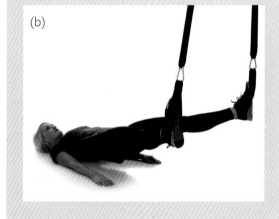

(b)

Target muscles: Gluteals, hamstrings, abductors and lumbar erectors
Technique rating: 1
Intensity rating: 2
Challenge rating: 3

Set-up
Straps anchored high and set at long range. Foot loops attached

Positioning
Begin lying face up with heels set in the foot loops, legs together and arms on the ground for stability

Quick guide
- Lift the hips off the ground until they are in alignment with the shoulders and heels in the loops and there is good spinal position
- Hold the reverse plank position while slowly moving the legs out wide and bringing them back together repeatedly
- Lower the hips back to the floor to bring the body to rest

Technical tips
- Keep the ankles, knees, hips, spine and shoulders in good alignment and as stable as possible during the reverse plank hold. The head should be relaxed and in contact with the ground throughout. Avoid looking up and flexing the neck
- The inward and outward movement of the legs should be fairly slow, smooth and controlled with neither the narrow or wide positions being held still
- As the core muscles begin to fatigue the body will tend to revert to its dominant postural position where it feels strongest, which may not always be in good spinal alignment. Avoid the pelvis rolling forwards and arching the lower back. Avoid twisting the spine as a result of one hip sagging lower than the other

Exercise 25 Suspended jackknife

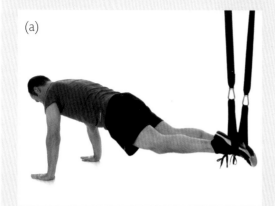

(a)

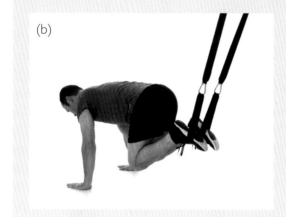

(b)

Target muscles: Abdominals
  and iliopsoas
Technique rating: 2
Intensity rating: 2
Challenge rating: 4

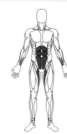

Set-up
Straps anchored high and set at long range. Foot loops attached

Positioning
Begin lying face down with feet set in the foot loops and elbows and forearms on the ground

Quick guide
- Lift the hips off the ground, push up on to the hands and hold the body in good alignment between the hands on the ground and feet suspended in the loops
- Bend the hips and knees drawing the legs under the body up towards the chest
- Keep the pelvis at a similar height as the shoulders throughout the whole movement
- Control the return movement, extending the hips and knees

Technical tips
- The jackknife requires a high degree of stabilisation through the torso and at the shoulder complex while simultaneously controlling movement at the legs
- As the straps are moving around a fixed anchor point they will arc upwards slightly lifting the feet in the loops as the knees are drawn under the body. This small upward motion should be compensated for through movement adjustment at the ankles, knees and hips. Upward movement of the pelvis to upset spinal alignment should be minimised or avoided if possible
- It is desirable to be able to draw the knees under the body through until the hips are beyond 90 degrees of flexion, ideally towards 120 degrees of flexion or thereabouts

Exercise 26 Suspended cycling jackknife

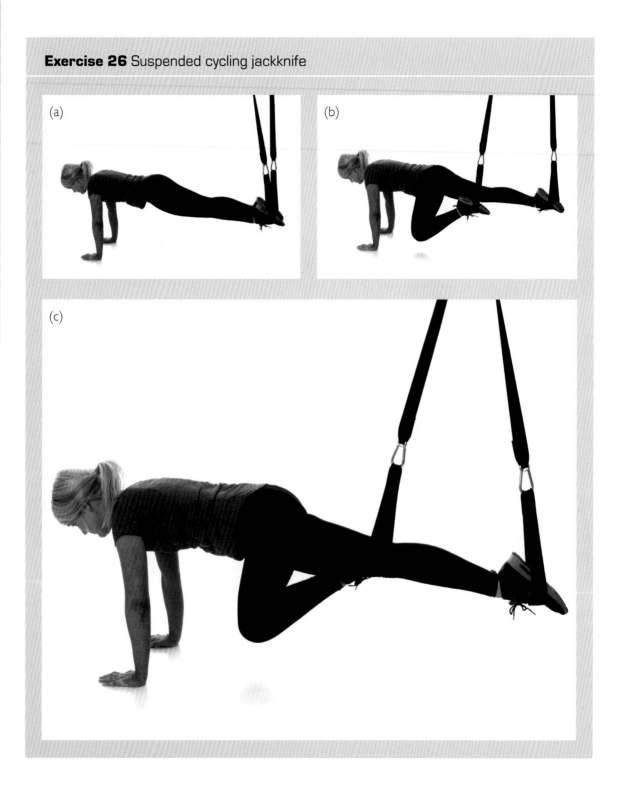

(a)

(b)

(c)

Target muscles: Abdominals
    and iliopsoas
Technique rating: 2
Intensity rating: 2
Challenge rating: 4

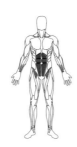

Set-up

Straps anchored high and set at long range. Foot loops attached

Positioning

Begin lying face down with feet set in the foot loops and elbows and forearms on the ground

Quick guide

- Lift the hips off the ground, push up on to the hands and hold the body in good alignment between the hands on the ground and feet suspended in the loops
- Bend the hip and knee of one leg drawing the knee under the body up towards the chest then return and repeat the same movement with the other leg and continue in a cyclical manner
- Keep the pelvis at a similar height as the shoulders throughout the whole movement cycle
- Control the speed of movement to be smooth and flowing without rapid, jerky actions

Technical tips

- The cycling jackknife requires a high degree of stabilisation through the torso and at the shoulder complex while simultaneously controlling the cyclical movement at the legs
- Cycling of the legs will create rotational forces up through the pelvis and spine. It is not expected that the torso will be held absolutely motionless, but the rotation of the spine should be kept to a minimum and maintained under some degree of control while the legs are moving
- Emphasis should be on drawing each leg in and out through a full range of motion with a smooth transition from one leg to the other, rather than on generating too much speed of movement

ADVANCED SUSPENDED EXERCISES

6

These more advanced exercises should not be attempted until you have mastered the basics. These exercises are too difficult for a keen individual to grasp, but they are progressing the basic exercises in the last chapter by adapting or adjusting the original technique. Exercise has a way of exposing weaknesses in physical capacity, technique or movement potential when the intensity or difficulty increases beyond an individual's current ability. Therefore, a solid understanding and full capacity to perform the basic exercises is essential. Once technique and form are strong enough it's time to take on the additional challenges in this chapter.

There are many different ways to increase the difficulty of suspended fitness training exercises. These include:

- Increasing the angle of loading so that gravitational pull on the target body part is more significant
- Altering the speed or momentum at which an exercise is to be performed, both slowing it down for greater time under tension and speeding it up for greater power and explosiveness
- Involving more body parts and joints so that exercise complexity and neural demand increases
- Drawing the straps forwards from the anchor point to increase the intensity of the pendulum effect
- Combining the movements from two or more exercises to create a more challenging compound exercise
- Altering the plane or direction of motion of the original exercise to vary the neural stimulus and adjust the original exercise technique that has been mastered
- Adding ground reaction and impact forces that require rapid control and proprioceptive responsiveness

The different exercises will still be organised into the same five movement patterns that were used in the previous chapter namely push, pull, squat, lunge and core control.

ADVANCED PUSH EXERCISES

Exercise 1 Alternating flye chest press

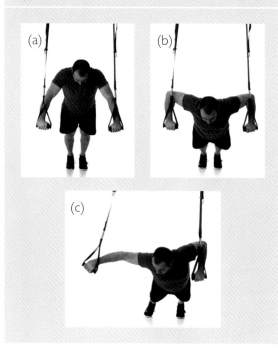

(a) (b) (c)

Target muscles: Pectorals, deltoids and triceps
Technique rating: 2
Intensity rating: 2
Challenge rating: 4

Set-up

Straps anchored high and set at equal length on each strap from mid to short. Standard handles attached

Positioning

Begin with the feet in a fixed neutral position behind the body and slightly in front of the anchor point. Face away from the anchor point and grip the handles close to either side of the chest just below shoulder height

Quick guide

- Lean forwards against the straps with elbows straight and keeping hands in front of shoulders
- Perform the first repetition as a standard chest press, returning to the start position
- The second repetition (shown in image c) requires that one arm is reached out wide, extending the elbow like a chest flye, whilst the other arm presses as normal
- Each repetition alternates between a normal chest press and a half press half flye variation
- Keep the chest lifted up and other key joints in good alignment throughout
- A full set may be done by only performing the flye repetitions on one arm e.g. left side only. This would be balanced out with right arm flyes during a full second set. Another option is to alternate the flye arm within a set e.g. 2 arm press, left arm flye, 2 arm press then right arm flye

Technical tips

- It is important to begin each press/flye motion with a shift of the flye arm out wide to the side of the body to maximise the activity of the pectorals and using the pressing arm to control and stabilise the descent. The return to the start position should follow the same path in reverse.
- It can be tempting to rotate the body towards the flye arm and let the better positioned pressing arm support the bulk of the load. The body needs to remain facing downwards and the angle of loading needs to be based on the workload that the flye arm can sustain without losing form

Exercise 2 Transverse chest press

(a)

(b)

(c)

(d)

Target muscles: Pectorals, deltoids and triceps
Technique rating: 2
Intensity rating: 2
Challenge rating: 4

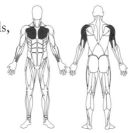

Set-up
Straps anchored high and set at equal length on each strap from mid to short. Standard handles attached

Positioning
Begin with feet in a neutral position wider than hip width apart and fixed behind the body but slightly in front of the anchor point. Face away from the anchor point and grip the handles with arms in front of the body at shoulder height

Quick guide
- Lean into the straps so that the arms take the load
- Bend at the elbows and shoulders, keeping the arms out wide bringing the body forward until chest is almost in line with handles
- Push back against the handles, driving one arm high and across the body to the other side and one arm low on the same side of the body until the arms are fully extended
- Draw the elbows back into the initial deep press position with chest forwards then repeat the press on the opposite side switching the low and high arms
- Repeat the press on alternating sides
- Keep the chest lifted up and other key joints in good alignment throughout

Technical tips
- Pressing one arm high and across the body draws the strap away from the anchor point, which is then be subject to the pendulum effect. This adds to the resistance felt against the higher pressing arm. Perform this in a slow and controlled manner to ensure an effective and safe press is performed on each side
- In order to press in the required directions with both arms, the spine needs to bend slightly towards the side with the low pressing arm. Spinal alignment in an anterior-posterior direction needs to remain strong

Exercise 3 High and wide chest flye

(a)

(b)

(c)

(d)

Target muscles: Pectorals
and deltoids
Technique rating: 2
Intensity rating: 3
Challenge rating: 5

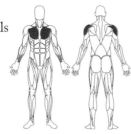

Set-up

Straps anchored high and set at equal length on each strap from mid to short. Standard handles attached

Positioning

Begin with feet placed in neutral stance and fixed behind the body but slightly anterior to the anchor point. Grip handles with the arms straight and in front of the body at shoulder level

Quick guide

- Lean into the straps so that the arms support the weight of the body
- Open one arm outwards in a wide lateral arc with the other arm simultaneously moving directly upwards into an overhead position, controlling the downward descent of the body at the same time
- Drive the wide arm forward and the high arm downward bringing the hands back in front of the body until they meet again in the middle
- Alternate the wide arm and high arm with each repetition
- Keep the chest lifted up and other key joints in good alignment

Technical tips

- Ensure that as the shoulders horizontally extend on one side and flex on the other that throughout the movement the wrist, elbow and shoulder joints are maintained in strict alignment with the elbow joint being kept slightly soft so it does not lock out
- Good joint and spinal alignment must be maintained throughout the press with ankles, knees, hips and spine all holding fixed to allow the body to form an effective lever that pivots on the ball of the foot during the flye movement
- Avoid the hips dropping forward with gravity or the body rotating towards the high side arm as this will place undue pressure on the lower back and increase injury risk
- The high arm shoulder is at some degree of risk if the load is excessive. It is important that the angle of the body overall is appropriate to ensure that the degree of body weight resistance being applied is matched by shoulder stability and strength. If the load is too great, move the feet forwards and fix them further away from the anchor point to reduce the load on the shoulder

Exercise 4 Stabilisation press-up

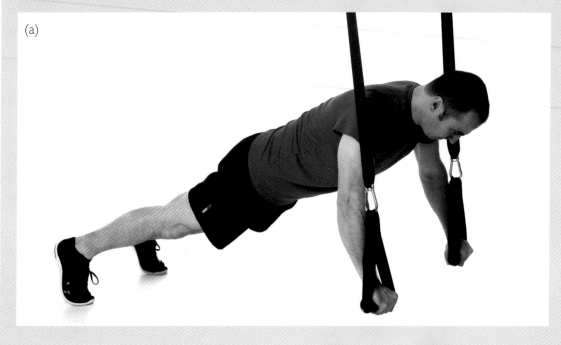

(a)

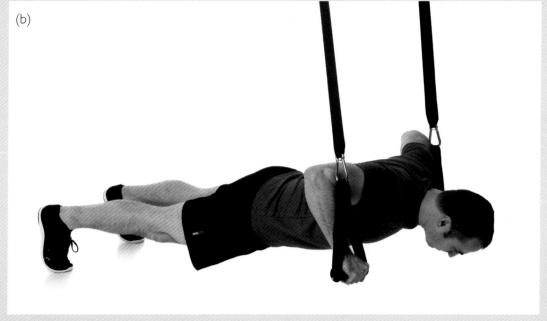

(b)

Target muscles: Pectorals,
   deltoids and triceps
Technique rating: 1
Intensity rating: 3
Challenge rating: 4

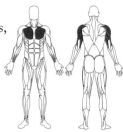

Set-up

Straps anchored high and set at equal length at long range. Handles attached

Positioning

Standard press-up position gripping the handles, arms locked out directly underneath the anchor point and feet together balancing on the toes

Quick guide

- Bend at the elbow and shoulders controlling the descent against gravity to lower the body down until the elbows are out to the sides at right angles, then drive upwards back to top position with the elbows locked out
- The small movements of the straps will need to be stabilised and corrected to maintain optimal position throughout the downward and upward movements of the press-up
- Hold the body in good alignment from feet to shoulders throughout each stabilisation press-ups

Technical tips

- This exercise will require the user to easily have the ability to perform full press-ups. Suspending the hands in the loops increases the load and difficulty of the exercise compared to normal press-ups by destabilising the shoulders which increases muscle activity all around the joint
- Avoid the hips dropping downward with gravity as this will place undue pressure on the lower back and increase spinal injury risk. Keep the ankles, knees, hips and shoulders in alignment parallel with the ground throughout each press-up
- Avoid rapidly descending or collapsing into the downward motion of the press-up as this may create unwanted movement of the straps and lead to collapse or injury. Strive to control the downward phase of the movement and transition smoothly into the upward press-up movement

Exercise 5 Stabilisation press-up to chest press

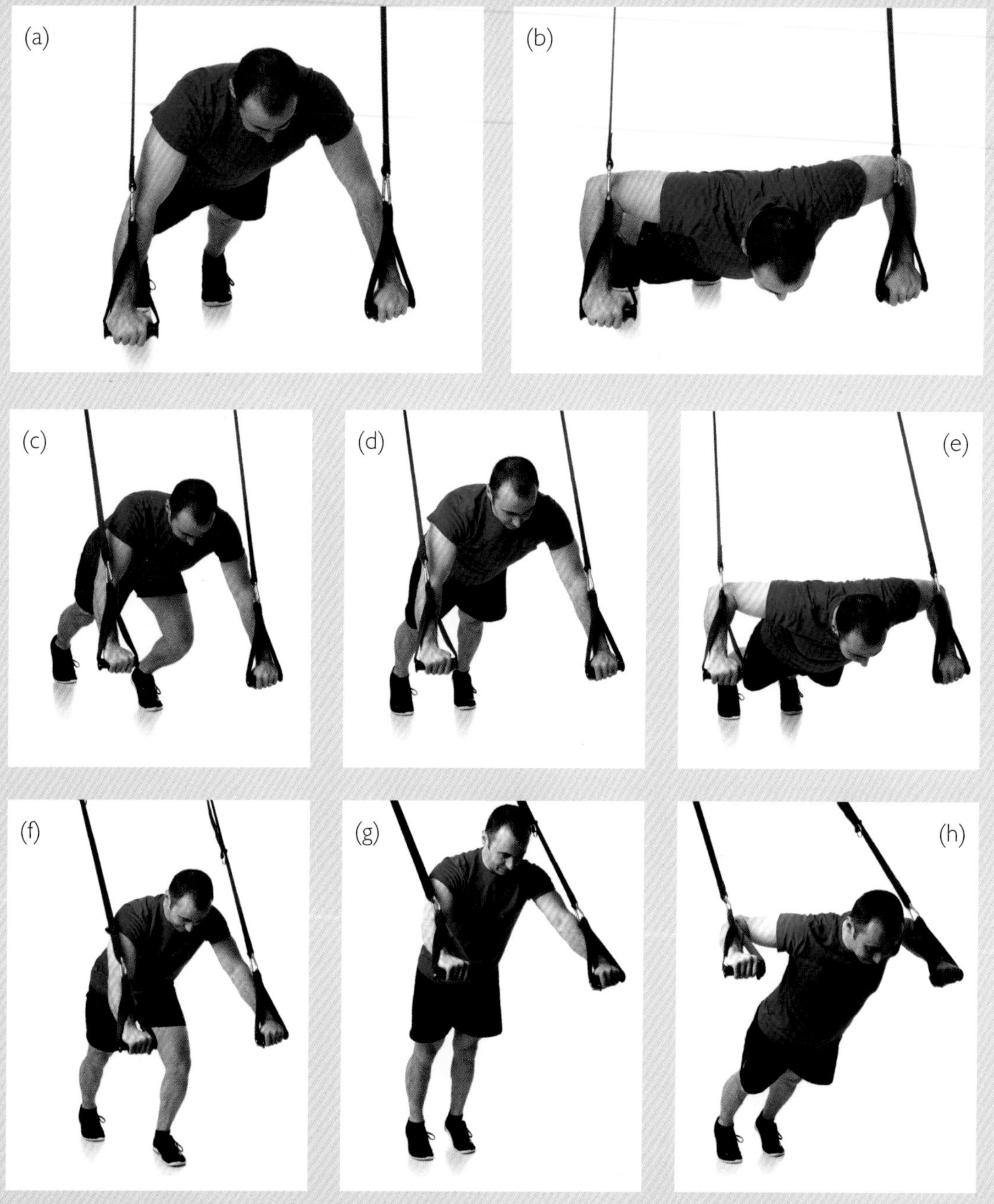

(a)

(b)

(c)

(d)

(e)

(f)

(g)

(h)

Target muscles: Pectorals, deltoids and triceps
Technique rating: 3
Intensity rating: 3
Challenge rating: 6

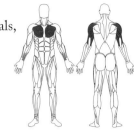

Set-up

Straps anchored high and set at equal length at long range. Handles attached

Positioning

Standard press-up position gripping the handles, arms locked out directly underneath the anchor point and feet together balancing on the toes

Quick guide

- Bend at the elbow and shoulders controlling the descent against gravity to lower the body down until the elbows are out to the sides at right angles, then drive upwards back to top position with the elbows locked out
- In between each press-up repetition while in a press-up plank position, step the legs forward about 6–8 inches to a new fixed point on the ground drawing the straps further forward then perform another press-up repetition. Each step forward and repetition will gradually bring the body from a face down press-up to a standing chest press
- Once the uppermost chest press position is reached the exercise should be performed in reverse to return back to the face down stabilisation press-up position
- The small movements of the straps will need to be stabilised and corrected to maintain optimal position throughout the downward and upward movements of the press-up

- Hold the body in good alignment from feet to shoulders throughout each stabilisation press-ups and chest press

Technical tips

- This exercise will require the user to easily have the ability to perform full press-ups. Suspending the hands in the loops increases the load and difficulty of the exercise compared to normal press-ups by destabilising the shoulders which increases muscle activity all around the joint
- The changing body angles alter the direction of strain and centre of gravity, varying the challenge with each press-up and chest press. Care needs to be taken to keep any wobble from the handles under control during each press
- Avoid dropping the hips downward with gravity as this will place undue pressure on the lower back and increase spinal injury risk. Keep the ankles, knees, hips and shoulders in alignment parallel with the ground throughout each press-up and chest press

Exercise 6 Walking suspended press-up

(a)

(b)

(c)

(d)

(e)

(f)

Target muscles: Pectorals, deltoids, triceps and abdominals

Technique rating: 2

Intensity rating: 3

Challenge rating: 5

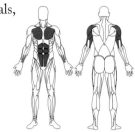

Set-up

Straps anchored high and set at equal length to long range. Foot loops attached

Positioning

Standard press-up position with hands flat on the ground, feet suspended with laces down in the foot loops and the feet directly underneath the anchor point

Quick guide

- Walk the arms forwards 2 to 3 steps drawing the straps forwards with the feet at the same time and resisting the pendulum pull effect that is created
- Bend at the elbow and shoulders controlling the descent against gravity to lower the body down until the elbows are out to the sides at right angles, then drive upwards back to top position with the elbows locked out
- Walk the arms backwards 2 or 3 steps to the start position, then repeat
- Hold the body in good alignment from feet to shoulders throughout each walking press-ups

Technical tips

- This exercise will require the user to already have the ability to perform full-suspended press-ups. Suspending the feet in the loops increases the load and difficulty of the exercise compared to normal press-ups by shifting a greater portion of body weight into the arms and by decreasing the stability of the body overall
- Avoid the hips dropping downward with gravity as this will place undue pressure on the lower back and increase spinal injury risk. Keep the ankles, knees, hips and shoulders in alignment parallel with the ground throughout each press-up
- The pendulum effect created by the forwards walk will intensify the work performed by the abdominals and iliopsoas muscles and will increase the chances of early fatigue which may lead to hips dropping down and excessive arching of the lower back. Poor form must not be allowed and the exercise must stop if hip and back form cannot be maintained
- Avoid rapidly descending or collapsing into the downward motion of the press-up. Strive to control the downward phase of the movement and transition smoothly into the upward press-up movement

Exercise 7 Multi-planar suspended press-up

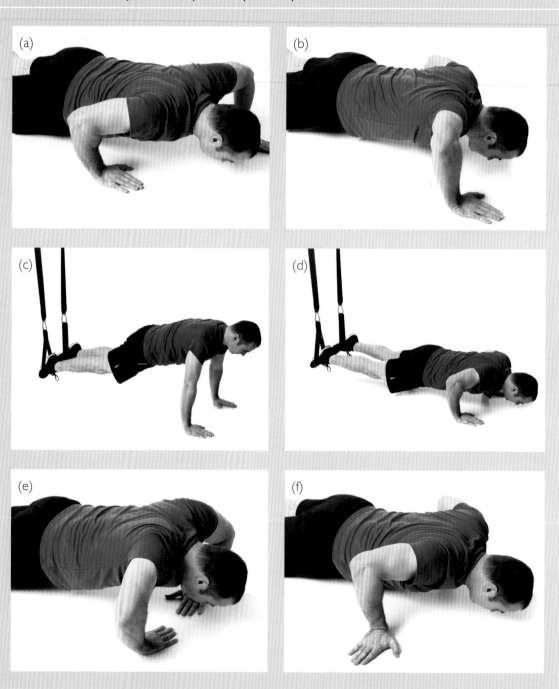

Target muscles: Pectorals, deltoids, triceps and abdominals
Technique rating: 2
Intensity rating: 3
Challenge rating: 5

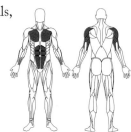

Set-up

Straps anchored high and set at equal length on each strap to long range. Foot loops attached

Positioning

Standard press-up position with hands flat on the ground, feet suspended laces down in the foot loops and the feet directly underneath the anchor point

Quick guide

- The key to this press-up variation is the 6 different hand positions that comprise one full cycle of repetitions:
  - Left hand high, right hand low
  - Right hand high, left hand low
  - Both hands narrow
  - Both hands wide
  - Both hands rotated inwards 90 degrees
  - Both hands rotated outwards 90 degrees
- Once each hand position is fixed in place, bend at the elbow and shoulders controlling the descent against gravity to lower the chest down towards the ground, then drive upwards back to top position with the elbows locked out
- Hold the body in good alignment from feet to shoulders throughout each press-up cycle

Technical tips

- This exercise will require the user to already have the ability to perform full-suspended press-ups. Suspending the feet in the loops increases the load and difficulty of the exercise compared to normal press-ups by shifting a greater portion of body weight into the arms and by decreasing the stability of the body overall
- Hand positions must only be changed at the top of each press-up move when the elbows are fully extended
- Avoid the hips dropping downward with gravity as this will place undue pressure on the lower back and increase spinal injury risk. Keep the ankles, knees, hips and shoulders in alignment parallel with the ground throughout each press-up
- Avoid rapidly descending or collapsing into the downward motion of the press-up. Each different hand position changes the mechanics of the press-up and may change the difficulty experienced from repetition to repetition. Strive to control the downward phase of the movement and transition smoothly into the upward press-up movement

Exercise 8 Inverted press

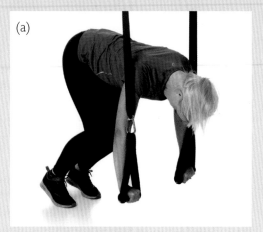

(a)

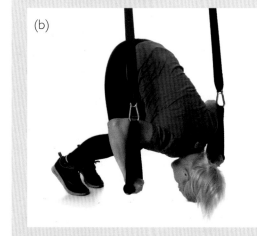

(b)

Target muscles: Deltoids and triceps
Technique rating: 2
Intensity rating: 2
Challenge rating: 4

Set-up
Straps anchored high and set at equal length to long range. Standard handles attached

Positioning
Begin with feet in neutral position directly under the anchor point, knees held straight and body bent at the hips in an inverted V position. Grip handles with arms outstretched overhead pointing to the floor

Quick guide
- Push up on to the toes and shift body weight slightly forward so that sufficient load is passed through the arms
- Bend at the elbows and shoulders to lower the body and move downward towards the ground in an inverse shoulder press
- Stop when the hands are level with the ears and drive the body upwards by pressing the arms back up into a straight position

Technical tips
- Body position must remain in the inverted V shape throughout the pressing motion and needs to pivot on the toes
- While a portion of total body weight will continue to pass through the feet the degree of difficulty will depend upon the centre of gravity shifting forwards over the hands holding the straps
- The hips must remain fully flexed with the knees extended throughout the press. Avoid the hips drifting out of flexion during the downward motion of the press as this will change the angle of loading on the shoulders and shift the work away from the deltoids and begin to involve the pectorals more
- The elbows must remain directly above the hands and the downward descent of the inverted press must be carefully controlled and stabilised to reduce risk of collapse at the shoulders or loss of control of the straps out wide

Exercise 9 Inverted wide press

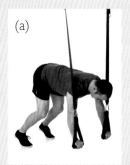
(a)

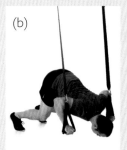
(b)

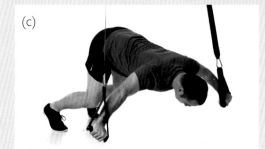
(c)

Target muscles: Deltoids and triceps
Technique rating: 2
Intensity rating: 3
Challenge rating: 5

Set-up
Straps anchored high and set at equal length to long range. Standard handles attached

Positioning
Begin with feet in neutral position directly under the anchor point, knees held straight and body bent at the hips in an inverted V position. Grip handles with arms outstretched overhead pointing to the floor.

Quick guide
- Push up on to the toes and shift body weight slightly forward so that sufficient load is passed through the arms
- Bend at the elbows and shoulders to lower the body and move downward towards the ground in an inverse shoulder press
- Stop when the hands are level with the ears and drive the body upwards by pressing the arms upward and out to the sides at 45 degrees
- Repeat each repetition under control

Technical tips
- Body position must remain in the inverted V shape throughout the pressing motion and needs to pivot on the toes
- While a portion of total body weight will continue to pass through the feet the degree of difficulty will depend upon a shift of centre of gravity forwards over the hands holding the straps. The wide inverted press will likely require a reduced load compared to the standard inverted press and the forward shift may not be as great
- The hips must remain fully flexed with the knees extended throughout the press. Avoid the hips drifting out of flexion during the downward motion of the press as this will change the angle of loading on the shoulders and shift the work away from the deltoids and begin to involve the pectorals more
- Each repetition of the wide inverted press must be carefully stabilised as the risk of technique failure and potential injury is higher than with the standard inverted press. As a means of progression it may be wise to start with a narrower pressing angle and working on strength and technique until the desired wider angle press can be achieved

ADVANCED PULL EXERCISES

Exercise 10 Supine wide arm pull-up

(a)

(b)

Target muscles: Mid-trapezius, rhomboids and deltoids
Technique rating: 1
Intensity rating: 3
Challenge rating: 4

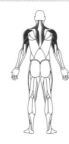

Set-up
Straps anchored high and set at equal length short- to mid-range. Standard handles attached

Positioning
Lie directly underneath the anchor point and grip handles at arm's length so that the body is lifted and the heels are the only body part making ground contact

Quick guide
- Pull upwards and wide driving the chest towards the anchor point
- Draw the elbows wide in line with the shoulders and squeeze the shoulder blades behind at the highest point of the pull
- Control the return to the start position and repeat
- Maintain body alignment from feet to shoulders throughout the exercise and pivot on the heels

Technical tips
- It helps to visualise pulling back from the elbows rather than the hands and driving them wide and back behind the body
- Drive the chest forward, lifting it up and towards the anchor point to help encourage full horizontal extension at the shoulder
- The lowering portion of the movement must be controlled and the return should be soft and smooth rather than jerky and bouncing
- Avoid the hips dropping downwards towards the ground as this tends to create momentum when initiating the movement, rather than the load being overcome only by the arms and back muscles

Exercise 11 Low to high straight-arm pull

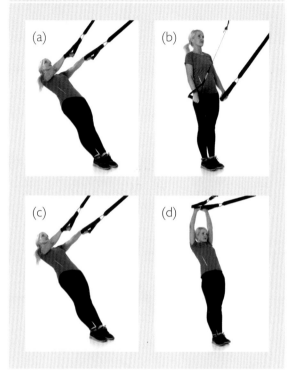

(a) (b) (c) (d)

Target muscles: Latissimus dorsi and deltoids
Technique rating: 3
Intensity rating: 2
Challenge rating: 5

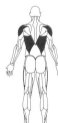

Set-up
Straps anchored high and set at equal length from short- to mid-range. Standard handles attached

Positioning
Feet are fixed slightly in front of the anchor point while facing towards the straps. Grip handles at arm's length and lean back to place straps under tension

Quick guide
- Quickly draw straight arms down and back until they are close to the sides of the body
- Immediately change direction controlling the return to the start position but flow past this point and drive the arms upwards until they are overhead in a straight position
- Control the return to the start position and repeat
- Keep body aligned from feet to shoulders throughout the exercise and pivot around the ankles or rock on the heels. Keep the chest lifted throughout.

Technical tips
- Keep the elbows extended and the arms strictly shoulder width apart throughout the downward and upward arm movements so that the primary driving movements are shoulder extension on the downward drive and shoulder flexion on the upward drive
- Avoid holding the arms static at the bottom of the downward drive or the top of the upward drive, but seek to flow under control from one position to the next
- Avoid the hips dropping downwards towards the ground as this tends to create momentum when initiating the movement, rather than the load being overcome only by the arms, shoulders and back musculature
- Keep the ankles, knees, hips and torso in alignment throughout each straight-arm pull, pivoting either at the ankle joint or rocking on the heel

Exercise 12 Hip thrust to row

(a)

(b)

(c)

Target muscles: Latissimus dorsi, biceps, deltoids and hamstrings
Technique rating: 2
Intensity rating: 2
Challenge rating: 4

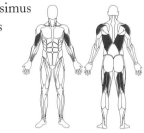

Set-up

Straps anchored high and set at equal length from short- to mid-range. Standard handles attached

Positioning

Begin with feet fixed slightly in front of the anchor point and face towards the straps. Grip handles at arm's length with straps under tension

Quick guide

- Bend at the hips lowering them towards the floor while keeping the chest lifted and the knees straight
- At the base of the movement powerfully drive the hips up and forwards while drawing the elbows behind the body keeping them tight into the sides
- Control the descent back to the low position with hips bent and arms straight
- Keep good alignment through the spine and other joints of the body

Technical tips

- When bending at the hips to lower into the start position it is important the knees remain extended. To aid this process it is easier to rock on the heels rather than keep the soles of the feet in contact with the ground. The shoulders and arms should naturally relax, moving into a straight arm overhead position
- The hip thrust and rowing movements should happen simultaneously by powerfully driving the hips upwards and the shoulders pulling back while allowing the elbows to flex as usual in a rowing action
- The upper finish position will create a straight aligned position from the ankles through to the shoulders with the elbows drawn back behind the body and tight to the sides of the lower ribs
- The positive pulling part of the movement should be performed powerfully whereas the negative part is lowered more slowly and under control back to the start position in readiness for the next repetition

Exercise 13 Hip thrust narrow row and reach

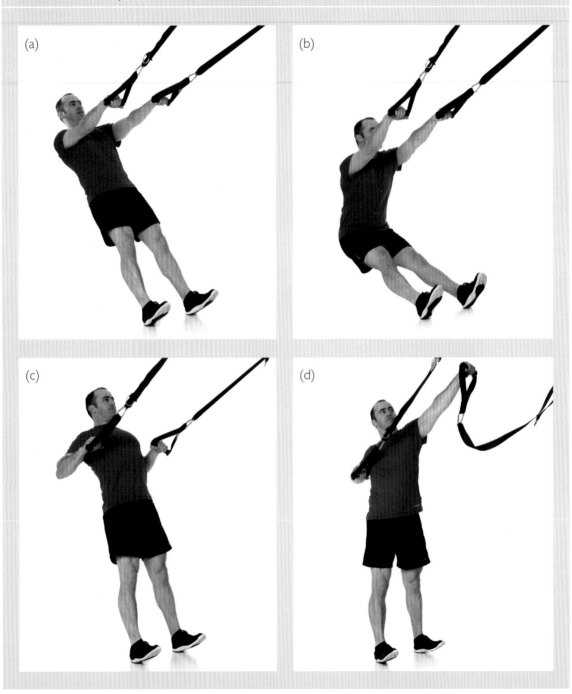

Target muscles: Latissimus
  dorsi, biceps and
  hamstrings
Technique rating: 3
Intensity rating: 2
Challenge rating: 5

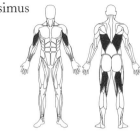

Set-up
Straps anchored high and set at equal length from short- to mid-range. Standard handles attached

Positioning
Begin with feet fixed wide and slightly in front of the anchor point and face towards the straps. Grip handles at arm's length with straps under tension.

Quick guide
- Bend at the hips, lowering them towards the floor while keeping the chest lifted and the knees straight
- At the base of the movement powerfully drive the hips up and forwards while pulling against the handle with a single arm, lifting the body up and drawing the elbow strongly behind the body while the other arm is quickly drawn forwards and reaches up towards the anchor point
- Allow the body to naturally rotate while reaching up with the free arm
- Control the descent back to the low position with hips bent and arms straight then repeat with the opposite arm performing the pull
- Keep good alignment through the spine and other joints of the body

Technical tips
- When bending at the hips to lower into the start position it is important the knees remain extended. To aid this process it is easier to rock on the heels rather than keep the soles of the feet in contact with the ground. The shoulders and arms should naturally relax moving into a straight arm overhead position.
- The hip thrust and rowing movements should happen simultaneously by powerfully driving the hips upwards and the shoulder pulling back while allowing the lead elbow to flex as usual in a rowing action. The speed of the upward pull must generate enough motion to reach the other arm high towards the anchor point, however the descent must be controlled and gravitational pull resisted
- Shoulder extension must be emphasised during the row to ensure the greatest load is created by the large latissimus dorsi muscle. Drawing the elbow and arm back towards the lower ribs and hip, rather than pulling the hand towards the shoulder, will help to achieve this

Exercise 14 Low pull to triceps press

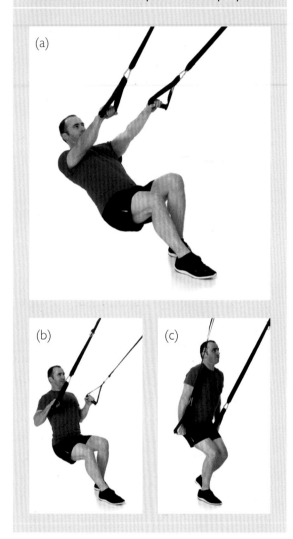

Set-up
Straps anchored high and set at equal length at mid-range. Standard handles attached

Positioning
Feet grounded in a split, partially weight-bearing position about 12–18 inches back from the anchor point and facing towards the straps. Grip handles at arm's length with straps under tension.

Quick guide
- Keep good alignment through spine and push hips back into a suspended half seating position
- Pull the elbows powerfully back behind and close to the sides of the body
- Drive the hips up and flow immediately into a low triceps extension with palms facing behind the body
- Control the reverse movement back to the start position

Technical tips
- Pulling the shoulders back needs to be a quick, powerful pulling motion to help create enough momentum to flow immediately into the tricep extension
- The driving hip extension phase should be timed to coincide with the start of the triceps extension as this will help to generate upward momentum and bring the repetition to its final position
- The positive or pulling part of the movement should be performed powerfully whereas the return must be lowered slowly and under control in readiness for the next repetition

Target muscles: Latissimus dorsi, biceps and triceps
Technique rating: 2
Intensity rating: 3
Challenge rating: 5

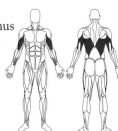

Exercise 15 Single arm wide row with single-leg squat

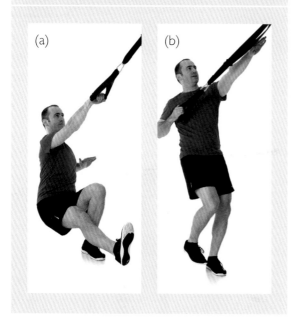

(a) (b)

Target muscles: Latissimus dorsi, biceps, quadriceps and gluteals
Technique rating: 3
Intensity rating: 3
Challenge rating: 6

Set-up
Straps anchored high and set at equal length at mid-range. Standard handles attached

Positioning
Begin standing on one leg with the other leg held slightly in front of the body. Grip one handle with the opposite arm to the stance leg and lean back so the strap is under tension

Quick guide
- Bend at the hip and knee of the stance leg to lower down into a deep single-leg squat position
- Drive the body upwards into a single leg standing position while simultaneously pulling against the strap so the elbow is drawn back wide at shoulder height, driving the chest forwards
- The free arm is moving opposite to the loaded arm at all times throughout the movement while the free leg is held out in front of the body with the knee straight
- Control the descent back to the start position and repeat

Technical tips
- The knee of the lead leg must remain over the first and second toes throughout the single-leg squat with the opposite leg being held straight out in front of the body
- The rotational forces that are created by standing on one leg and controlling with the opposite arm must be stabilised and controlled to allow for the desired movement during the exercise
- When the pulling arm is drawn back at shoulder level the opposite arm is reaching forwards in front of the body and vice versa. The opposing arm movements will help drive the rotation of the torso and aid in maintaining balance

ADVANCED SQUAT EXERCISES

Exercise 16 Lateral squat jump

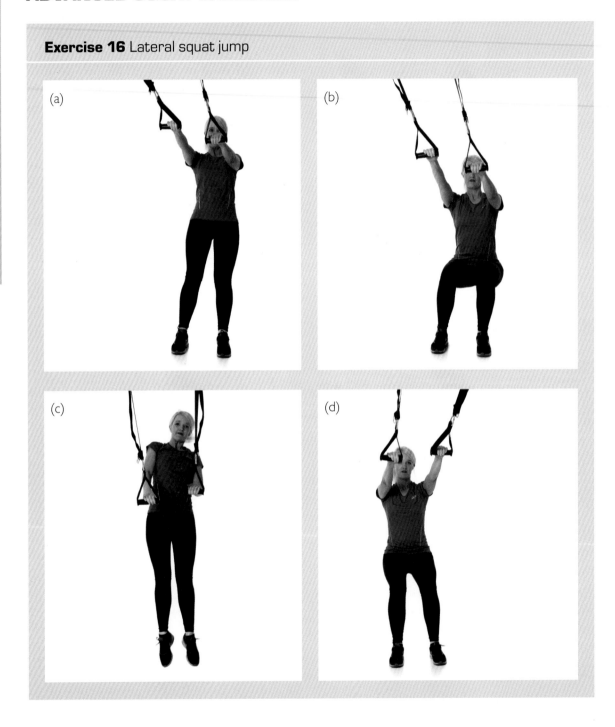

Target muscles:
   Quadriceps, gluteals
   and calf complex
Technique rating: 1
Intensity rating: 3
Challenge rating: 4

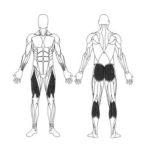

Set-up

Straps anchored high and set at equal length from short- to mid-range. Standard handles attached

Positioning

Begin with feet fixed in a neutral position approximately 18–24 inches (45–60 cm) in front of and to the left of the anchor point. Face the anchor point and grip the handles at arm's length leaning back to create tension in the straps

Quick guide

- Bend at the hips and quickly lower the body downwards while simultaneously bending at the knees until a squat position is reached with knees and hips close to right angles
- Drive the legs powerfully upwards and to the right, moving laterally in the air, landing again softly on the balls of the feet to then return back to the squat position
- Repeat the lateral jump immediately moving from the right to the left side
- Keep the arms at full length and lean back against the straps throughout the lateral squat jump movement so that they can provide a degree of balance
- Keep the chest lifted and shoulders drawn back throughout the movement

Technical tips

- It is important that the motion created by the jump creates a considerable amount of sideways travel in the air. A small sideways jump with good height is not the intention, but a strong sideways countermovement that loads the outer leg in the frontal plane to a greater degree is the objective
- Avoid excessive flexing at the hips in the downward loading phase of the movement where the angle of the spine exceeds the angle of the tibia at the lowest point of the movement. However, some frontal loading of the hips is desirable and may highlight differences in ability in terms of left and right side technique and performance

Exercise 17 Transverse squat jump

(a)

(b)

(c)

(d)

Target muscles:
Quadriceps, gluteals
and calf complex
Technique rating: 2
Intensity rating: 3
Challenge rating: 5

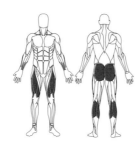

Set-up
Straps anchored high and set at equal length from short- to mid-range. Standard handles attached

Positioning
Begin with feet fixed in a neutral position approximately 18–24 inches (45–60 cm) in front of and to the left of the anchor point. Face to the left 45-60 degrees away from the anchor point and grip the handles at arm's length leaning back to create tension in the straps

Quick guide
- Bend at the hips and quickly lower the body downwards while simultaneously bending at the knees until a squat position is reached with knees and hips close to right angles
- Drive the legs powerfully upwards and rotate towards the right, travelling over the ground left to right while rotating body position 90–120 degrees in the air, landing again softly on the balls of the feet in a position 45–60 degrees facing away to the right of the anchor point
- Repeat the transverse jump immediately rotating in the air from the right to the left side
- Keep the arms positioned to retain the tension in the straps throughout the transverse squat jump, though this will require that the arms rotate in the opposite direction in relation to the body

- Keep the chest lifted and shoulders drawn back throughout the movement

Technical tips
- It is important that the motion created by the jump creates a considerable amount of sideways and rotational travel. A small rotational jump with good height is not the intention, but strong rotational countermovement that loads the outer leg in the transverse plane to a greater degree is the objective
- Avoid excessive flexing at the hips in the downward loading phase of the movement where the angle of the spine exceeds the angle of the tibia at the lowest point of the movement. However, some transverse loading of the hips is desirable as internal hip rotation is an effective movement that can generate good power output
- Care must be taken to ensure rotation is occurring at the hip and not the lumbar spine. Restrictions in hip motion may be compensated for by increased rotation at the spine which increases injury risk. Effective warm-up and hip mobility is desirable before performance of this exercise

Exercise 18 Single-leg squat jump

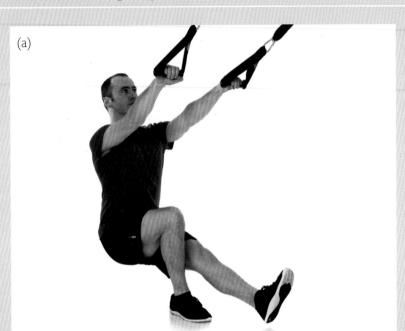

(a)

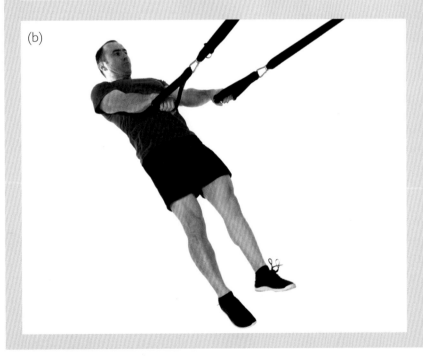

(b)

Target muscles:
Quadriceps, gluteals and calf complex

Technique rating: 2
Intensity rating: 4
Challenge rating: 6

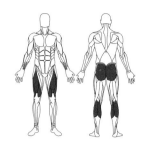

Set-up
Straps anchored high and set at short- to mid-range. Standard handles attached

Positioning
Begin facing towards the anchor point in a standing single-leg balance position with the non-standing leg held slightly in front of the body. The handles are held at arm's length, leaning back slightly with the straps under tension

Quick guide
- Bend the hip and knee of the stance leg to quickly lower the body down into a single-leg squat
- The non-weight-bearing leg is held off the ground out in front of the body during the squat-loading phase
- Powerfully drive upwards to jump vertically into the air, the trail leg being allowed to lower down alongside the jumping leg during the upward phase of motion
- Land softly through the ball of the foot on the lead leg and regain balance, then repeat
- Keep good spinal alignment while holding the handles at arm's length and maintaining tension in the straps throughout

Technical tips
- The single-leg squat jump requires much more conscious focus on maintaining balance both during the loading and landing phases of the exercise. Keeping tension through the straps will help maintain balance and control during the exercise.
- Ensure the chest is kept lifted and spinal alignment is maintained during the squat jump.
- While a high, explosive squat jump is desirable it should not come at the expense of a loss of form, especially compensations like sideways knee collapse or forward flexion of the spine.

Exercise 19 Single-leg frontal squat jump

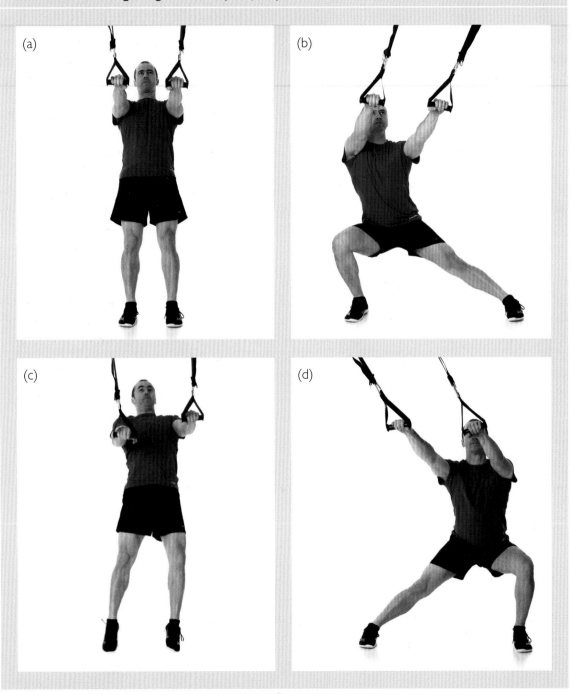

Target muscles:
   Quadriceps, gluteals,
   adductors and
   calf complex

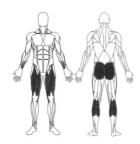

Technique rating: 2
Intensity rating: 4
Challenge rating: 6

Set-up

Straps anchored high and set at short- to mid-range. Standard handles attached

Positioning

Begin positioned to the left of the anchor point in a standing single-leg balance position with the non-standing leg held slightly in front of the body. The handles are held at arm's length, leaning back slightly with the straps under tension

Quick guide

- Bend the hip and knee of the stance leg to quickly lower the body down into a partial depth single-leg squat
- The non-weight-bearing leg is held off the ground out in front of the body during the squat loading phase
- Powerfully drive upwards to jump vertically and across to the right side, the trail leg being allowed to drop down alongside the jumping leg during the upward/travelling phase of motion
- Land softly through the ball of the foot on the lead leg and regain balance, then repeat by jumping back across to the left side
- Keep good spinal alignment while holding the handles at arm's length and maintaining tension in the straps throughout

Technical tips

- The single-leg squat jump requires much more conscious focus on maintaining balance both during the loading and landing phases of the exercise. Keeping tension through the straps will help maintain balance and control during the exercise
- Ensure the chest is kept lifted and spinal alignment is maintained during the squat jump
- While a high, explosive frontal squat jump is desirable it should not come at the expense of a loss of form, especially compensations like sideways knee collapse which is a greater risk during a sideways squat jump
- Once the single-leg frontal squat jump has been mastered with a pause between each jump to rebalance, the exercise can be performed without any pause where the intention is to immediately reload upon landing using the downward momentum to drop back into a single-leg squat and explode back into the next jump without any pause. Note: This rapid bounding jump progression is a high-intensity, high-impact exercise

Exercise 20 Single-leg transverse squat jump

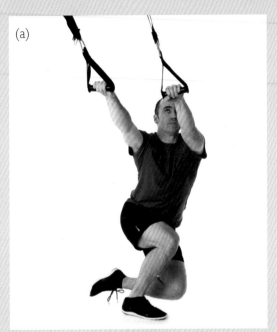

(a)

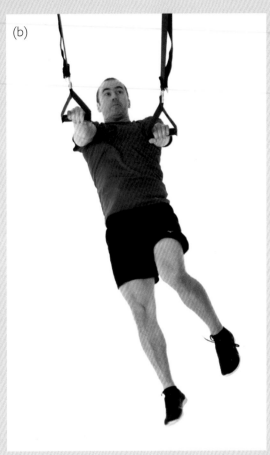

(b)

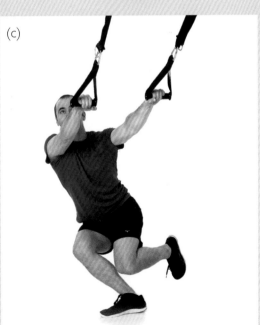

(c)

Target muscles:
  Quadriceps, gluteals,
  adductors and
  calf complex
Technique rating: 3
Intensity rating: 4
Challenge rating: 7

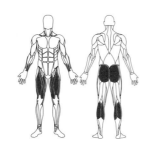

Set-up
Straps anchored high and set at short- to mid-range. Standard handles attached

Positioning
Begin facing 45 degrees away on the left side of the anchor point in a standing single-leg balance position with the non-standing leg held slightly in front of the body. The handles are held at arm's length, leaning back slightly with the straps under tension

Quick guide
- Bend the hip and knee of the stance leg to quickly lower the body down into a partial depth single-leg squat
- The non-weight-bearing leg is held off the ground out in front of the body during the squat loading phase
- Powerfully drive upwards to jump vertically and across to the right side, rotating the body approximately 90 degrees, the trail leg being allowed to drop down alongside the jumping leg during the upward/travelling phase of motion
- Land softly through the ball of the foot on the lead leg and regain balance, then repeat by jumping back across and rotating 90 degrees back to the left side

- Keep good spinal alignment while holding the handles at arm's length and maintaining tension in the straps throughout

Technical tips
- The single-leg transverse squat jump requires much more conscious focus on maintaining balance both during the loading and landing phases of the exercise. Keeping tension through the straps will help maintain balance and control during the exercise
- Ensure the chest is kept lifted and spinal alignment is maintained during the transverse squat jump
- While a high, explosive transverse squat jump is desirable it should not come at the expense of a loss of form, especially compensations like sideways or rotational knee collapse which is a greater risk due to the rotational nature of this exercise
- Once the transverse squat jump has been mastered with a pause between each jump to rebalance, the exercise can be performed without any pause where the intention is to immediately reload upon landing using the downward momentum to drop back into a transverse single-leg squat and explode back into the next jump without any pause. Note: This rapid bounding jump progression is a high intensity, high impact exercise

ADVANCED LUNGE EXERCISES

Exercise 21 Suspended lunge with multi-directional reach

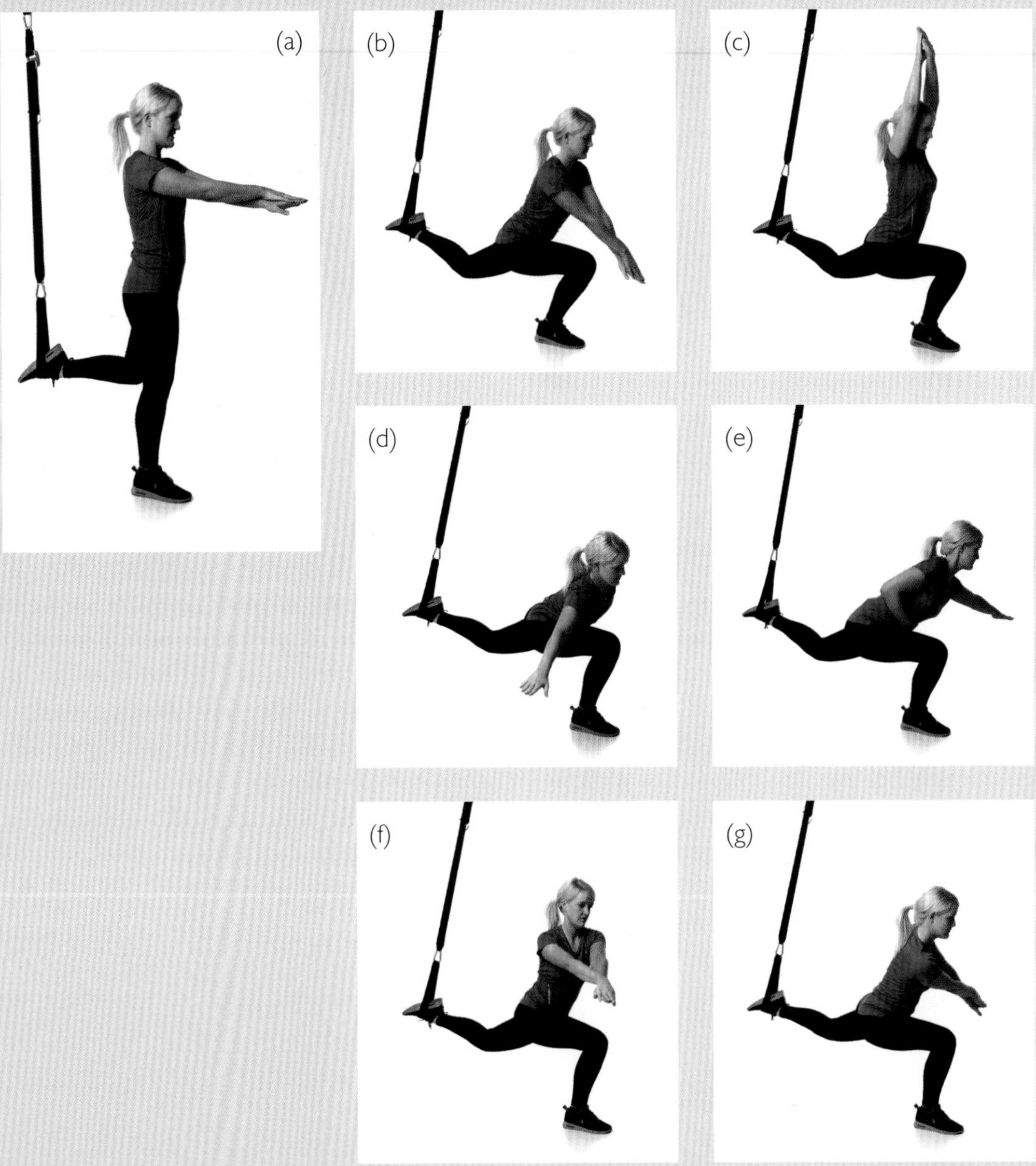

(a)

(b)

(c)

(d)

(e)

(f)

(g)

Target muscles: Gluteals, quadriceps, abductors and calf complex

Technique rating: 3

Intensity rating: 2

Challenge rating: 5

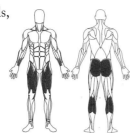

Set-up

Strap anchored high and set at full length. A foot loop should be attached

Positioning

A single foot is fixed to the ground in a neutral position about 3 feet in front of and facing away from the anchor point. The other foot is placed in the foot loop attached to the strap with the sole of the foot facing upwards

Quick guide

- Move forward so that the rear foot in the loop pulls the strap forward a little
- Bend at the stance leg knee and hip to move the body downward, dropping into a deep lunge position
- Drive back up to the start position. Add in arm reaches for variation with each repetition. Once a full set is completed repeat the exercise but switch legs
- Reach the arms in six different directions with each lunge repetition to challenge the lead leg and create variable muscular activation
  - Two hand anterior low reach
  - Two hand posterior overhead reach
  - One hand outside low reach
  - One hand inside low reach
  - Two hand external rotational reach
  - Two hand internal rotational reach

Technical tips

- Maintaining balance during this exercise may be a challenge in the early stages especially when the muscles involved are beginning to fatigue after a number of repetitions and stabilisation at the joint becomes less controlled. Care should be taken to prevent unwanted falls by exercising near a wall, chair or other object to secure oneself if needed
- The variety of different arm reaches will create different loading patterns for the muscles that control the ankle, knee and hip. The low anterior, low inside and external rotational reaches will all increase hip muscle activation in different planes of motion, whereas the posterior overhead, low outside and internal rotational reaches will reduce hip muscle activation and require greater muscle activation from other muscles controlling the knee and ankle
- The knee of the lead leg should remain over the first and second toes during the anterior and posterior reaching lunges. The side and rotational reaching lunges will alter loading patterns and the knee will not remain over the first and second toes, but will play a part in counterbalancing the forces being passed through the body
- This exercise can also be performed as a frontal lunge reaching pattern. The trail leg is held straight with knee extended and the foot in the loop out to the side of the body. The stance leg lunges would be performed with arm reaches following the same multi-directional pattern

Exercise 22 Suspended jump lunge

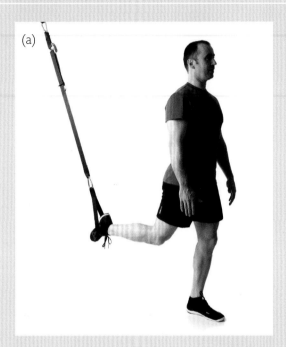

(a)

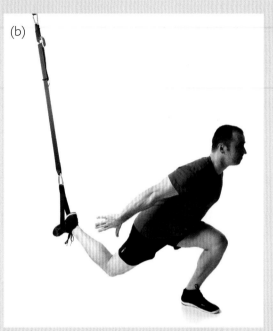

(b)

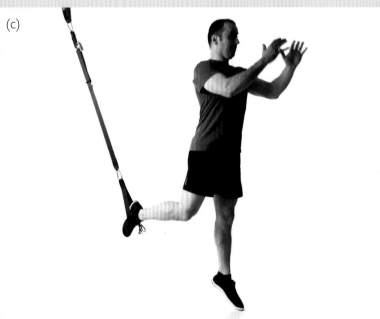

(c)

Target muscles: Gluteals, quadriceps and calf complex
Technique rating: 2
Intensity rating: 4
Challenge rating: 6

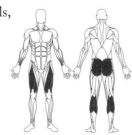

Set-up

Strap anchored high and set at full length. A foot loop should be attached

Positioning

A single foot is fixed to the ground in a neutral position about 3 feet in front of and facing away from the anchor point. The other foot is placed in the foot loop attached to the strap with the sole of the shoe facing upwards

Quick guide

- Move forward so that the rear foot in the loop pulls the strap forward at an angle
- Bend at the stance leg knee and hip to move the body quickly downward, loading the joints and muscles in a partial depth lunge position
- Reach the arms down and behind the body to help load the muscles
- Powerfully drive the lead leg upwards while simultaneously driving the arms forwards and upwards jumping vertically into the air.
- Land softly on the ball of the foot, regain balance and then repeat

Technical tips

- Maintaining balance during this exercise may be a challenge especially when landing after each jump and when the muscles involved are beginning to fatigue after a number of repetitions and stabilisation at the joint becomes less controlled. If needed perform the exercise near a wall, chair or another object to provide balance
- When performing the suspended jumping lunge it is acceptable to bend more at the hip than at the ankle. The powerful hip musculature are vital in creating upward force, however where joint range is available maximal movement at the ankle should be used to assist in vertical lift
- Well-timed back and forwards arm drive will help significantly in creating a whole-body loading and exploding pattern and improve vertical lift
- The knee of the lead leg knee move over the first and second toes during both the drive phase and landing phase of the jumping lunge

Exercise 23 Hanging frontal jump lunge

(a)

(b)

(c)

(d)

Target muscles:
  Quadriceps, abductors
  and gluteals
Technique rating: 3
Intensity rating: 3
Challenge rating: 6

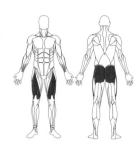

Set-up

Straps anchored high and set at mid-range. Standard handles attached

Positioning

Start in a standing wide-stance position with body weight shifted over the left leg. The handles are held at arm's length facing towards the anchor point, leaning back with the straps under tension

Quick guide

- Quickly bend the knee and hip of the left leg to lower into a loaded lunge position
- Drive powerfully with the left leg upward and across to the right side, switching sides with a quick crossover step to land softly on the right-hand side with the right leg bent in the lead lunge position
- Keep good spinal alignment throughout and maintain good knee alignment during alternate lunge loading and jumping phases

Technical tips

- The lead leg should always be the outermost leg for each lunge jump as the body moves across from side to side (i.e., the left leg leads for the loading and jumping phases on the left side and vice versa)
- While some vertical height is desirable for each lunge jump the objective is cover a good sideways distance while travelling from the left to right sides and back again. Emphasising sideways motion will help load the hips knees and ankles in the frontal plane
- It may be necessary upon landing to pause momentarily to regain balance before carrying out the next repetition. Once this has been mastered the exercise can be performed without any pause between repetitions where the downward momentum of landing immediately loads the opposite leg lunge ready for the next jumping repetition

Exercise 24 Hanging ice skater

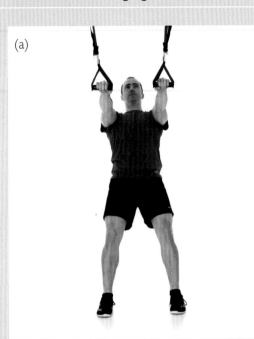

(a)

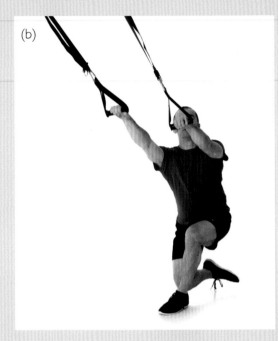

(b)

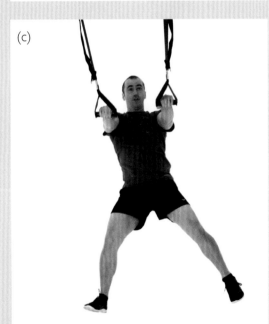

(c)

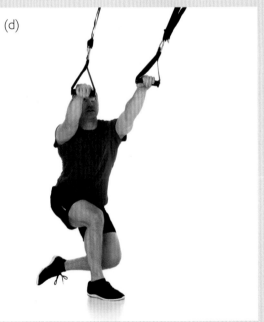

(d)

Target muscles:
Quadriceps, abductors
and gluteals
Technique rating: 3
Intensity rating: 4
Challenge rating: 7

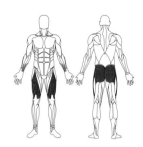

Set-up

Straps anchored high and set at mid-range. Standard handles attached

Positioning

Start in a standing wide-stance position with body weight shifted over the leg. The handles are held at arm's length facing towards the anchor point, leaning back with the straps under tension

Quick guide

- Quickly bend the knee and hip of the left leg to lower into a loaded lunge position with the trail leg lifted off the ground
- Drive powerfully with the left leg across to the right side, jumping in the air to land softly on the right-hand side with the right leg
- Using momentum immediately load back into the right leg quickly bending the hip and knee with the trail leg lifted off the ground, then powerfully jump back across to the left side
- Seek to maintain good knee alignment during alternate side-lunge loading and jumping phases
- When jumping off the left leg simultaneously pull the body across with the right arm strap and vice versa

Technical tips

- While some vertical height is desirable for each ice-skater drive, the objective is to powerfully travel sideways from left to right and back again. Emphasising sideways motion will help load the hips knees and ankles in the frontal plane
- The intention is to rapidly jump from leg to leg without any delay. Using the opposite leg and arm together to stabilise and decelerate motion upon landing to then drive motion into the next jump will aid quick and purposeful movement
- Care must be taken that the trail leg does not swing to rapidly from side to side such that it creates a rotational force when landing that will load the joints incorrectly and twist the knee increasing injury risk

Exercise 25 Hanging transverse jump lunge

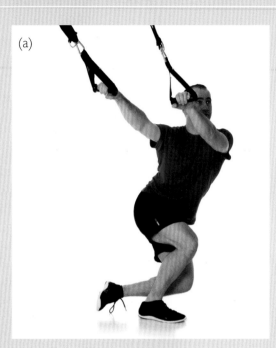

(a)

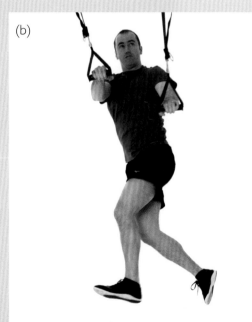

(b)

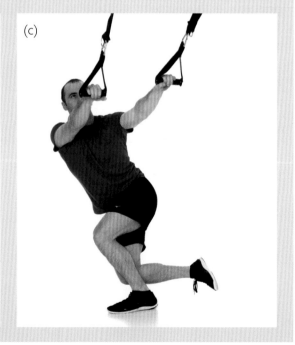

(c)

Target muscles: Gluteals, calf complex, quadriceps and obliques
Technique rating: 4
Intensity rating: 3
Challenge rating: 7

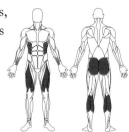

Set-up

Straps anchored high and set at mid-range. Standard handles attached.

Positioning

Start in a standing, neutral stance position. The handles are held at arm's length facing towards the anchor point, leaning back with the straps under tension.

Quick Guide

- Step the right leg inside and across the left leg to the left side placing the right foot on the ground in a 90° internally rotated position
- Quickly lunge down bending the right side hip and knee
- Drive powerfully with the right leg upward and across to the right side, switching sides with a quick crossover step to land softly on the right hand side with the left leg in the lead lunge position and left foot internally rotated 90°
- Keep good spinal alignment throughout and maintain good knee alignment over the lead foot during alternate transverse lunge loading and jumping phases

Technical Tips

- The lead leg should always be the forward leg for each lunge jump as the body moves across from side to side (i.e. the right leg leads for the loading and jumping phases on the left side and vice versa)
- Whilst some vertical height is desirable for each lunge jump the objective is to cover a good sideways distance while travelling from the left to right sides and back again. Emphasising rotational motion will help load the hips and obliques in the transverse plane.
- It may be necessary upon landing to pause momentarily to regain balance before carrying out the next repetition. Once this has been mastered the exercise can be performed without any pause between repetitions where the downward momentum of landing immediately loads the lead leg ready for the next jumping repetition

Exercise 26 Jumping sprint start

(a)

(b)

Target muscles:
Quadriceps, calf complex
and gluteals
Technique rating: 2
Intensity rating: 4
Challenge rating: 6

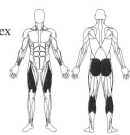

Set-up

Straps anchored high and set at mid-range. Standard handles attached

Positioning

Start in a deep split-lunge position facing away from the anchor point and leaning forward into the handles. Handles are held close to the body on either side of the chest

Quick guide

- Powerfully drive forward and up into the air using the lead or forward leg
- Simultaneously draw the trail leg through and drive the knee up and forwards in front of the body
- Keep good spinal alignment while continuously leaning forward into the straps with handles remaining close to sides of the chest so that the body swings in an arc upward with the straps
- Swing back, land softly and control the descent returning the trail leg to the ground behind and lowering the body by bending the hip and knee of the lead leg back to the start
- After a completed set, repeat with opposite leg leading the exercise

Technical tips

- The forward leaning position required in this exercise increases the work carried out by muscles surrounding the leading ankle and knee while relatively less work is performed by the hip musculature
- The primary focus of this exercise is to drive hard and reach maximal vertical height in a forward leaning sprint position
- It may be necessary upon landing to pause momentarily to regain balance before carrying out the next repetition. Once this has been mastered the exercise can be performed without any pause between repetitions where the downward momentum of landing immediately loads the lead leg lunge for the next jumping repetition

ADVANCED CORE EXERCISES

Exercise 27 Suspended body saw

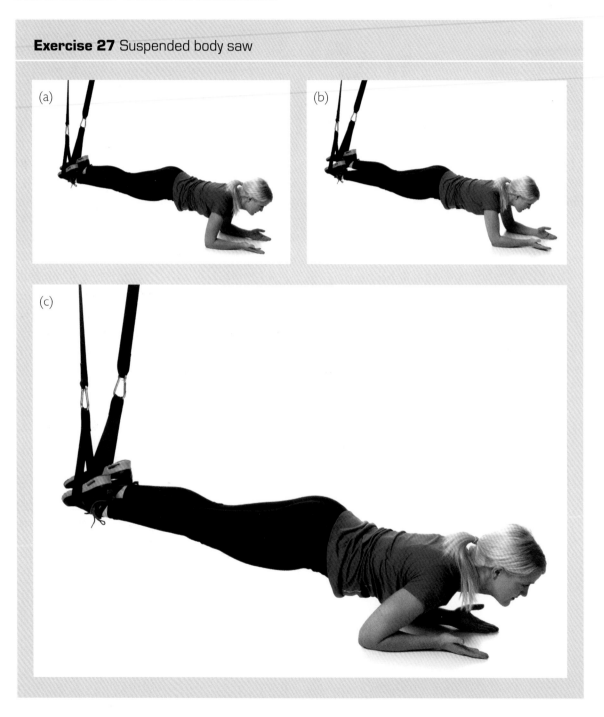

Target muscles: Abdominals
   and iliopsoas
Technique rating: 1
Intensity rating: 3
Challenge rating: 4

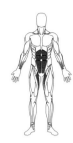

Set-up
Straps anchored high and set at long range. Foot
loops attached

Positioning
Begin lying face down with feet set in the foot
loops and elbows and forearms on the ground

Quick guide
- Lift the hips off the ground until they are in
  alignment with the shoulders and feet in the
  loops and there is good spinal position
- While maintaining hip alignment draw the
  body forwards over the fixed-arm position
  and then push backwards to extend the arms
  beyond the head
- Repeat this rocking motion to resemble a
  sawing action
- Once the repetitions are completed, lower the
  hips and torso to the floor to bring the body
  to rest

Technical tips
- Keep the ankles, knees, hips, spine and shoulders in good alignment and as stable as possible
  during the exercise. The head should also be in
  line with the eyes looking directly at the ground.
  Avoid looking up and extending the neck
- The sawing motion is generated by the arms
  only and the shoulder and elbows should be
  the only joints moving, the rest of the body is
  kept stable
- The sawing action will bring the pendulum
  effect into play and the intensity of the exercise is much greater than a standard suspended
  plank
- As the core muscles begin to fatigue the body
  will tend to revert to its dominant postural
  position where it feels strongest, which is often
  not optimal plank position. Avoid the pelvis
  tilting forwards and arching of the lower back.
  Avoid excessive mid-back curvature or the hips
  raised high out of alignment. Avoid pelvic rotation where one side of the body or one hip sags
  lower than the other
- Cease the exercise if good spinal position
  cannot be maintained

Exercise 28 Suspended superman

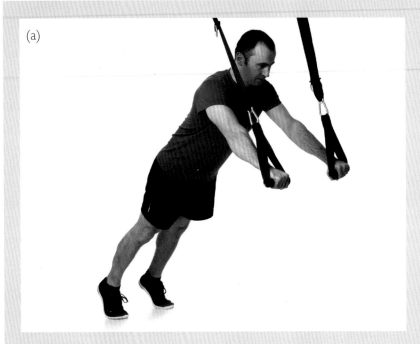

(a)

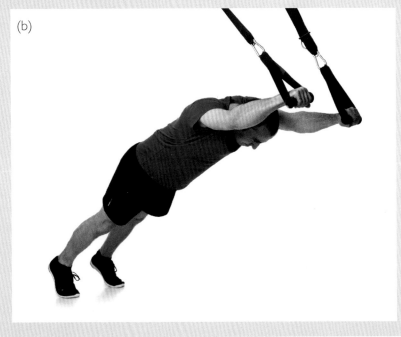

(b)

Target muscles:
Abdominals, iliopsoas and latissimus dorsi
Technique rating: 1
Intensity rating: 3
Challenge rating: 4

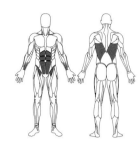

Set-up

Straps anchored high and set at short to medium range. Handles attached

Positioning

Begin standing in a neutral stance directly under the anchor point holding the handles just in front of hips

Quick guide

- Lean forward and using the handles to support body weight, control the descent of the body as the arms are raised directly overhead
- Maintain good alignment seeking to create a straight line from ankles to hands if possible where physical strength is sufficient
- Draw the arms downwards and back towards the hips to help bring the body back to a standing position

Technical tips

- Keep the ankles, knees, hips, spine and shoulders in good alignment and as stable as possible during the exercise. The head should also be in line with the eyes looking directly forwards. Avoid looking up and extending the neck
- The only joint in the body that should be moving during this exercise is the shoulders which are moving the arms up into flexion as the body descends and then back downwards as the body rises again

- The shoulders are under a lot of strain to control the movement associated with this exercise which increases the lower down the body travels. While the goal is to create a straight body line, this may be too difficult for some and as the shoulder range must remain within controllable extremes
- As the core muscles begin to fatigue the body will tend to revert to its dominant postural position where it feels strongest, which is often not optimal alignment. Avoid the pelvis tilting forwards and arching of the lower back. Avoid excessive mid-back curvature or the hips raised high out of alignment. Avoid pelvic rotation where one side of the body or one hip sags lower than the other
- Cease the exercise if good spinal position cannot be maintained

Exercise 29 Suspended walking plank

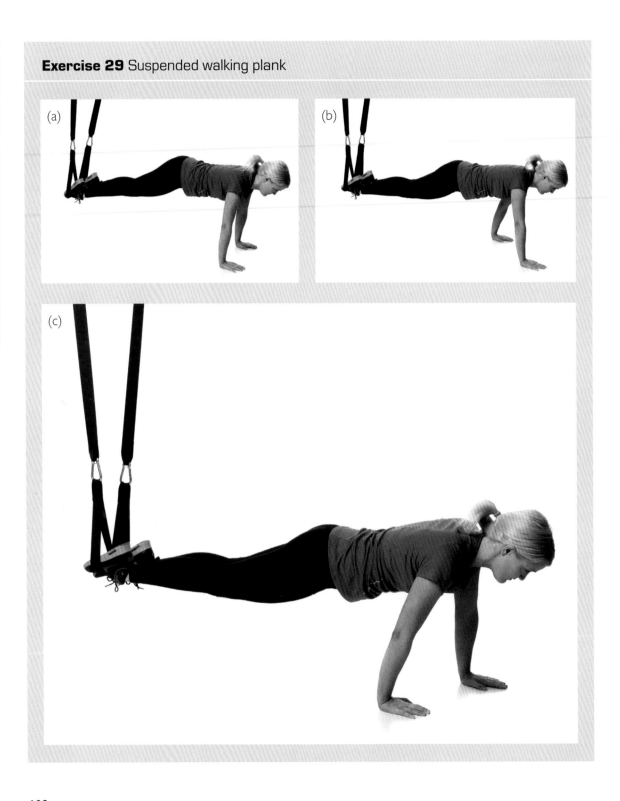

Target muscles:
Abdominals, iliopsoas
and deltoids
Technique rating: *2*
Intensity rating: *3*
Challenge rating: *5*

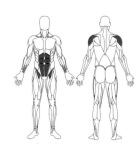

Set-up
Straps anchored high and set at long range. Foot loops attached

Positioning
Begin lying face down with feet set in the foot loops and elbows and forearms on the ground

Quick guide
- Lift the hips off the ground and push up off the elbows on to the hands with elbows locked out. Keep hips in alignment with the shoulders and feet in the loops and there is good spinal position
- While maintaining good hip alignment walk the hands forward a few steps which in turn will draw the straps forward, then return by walking the hands back to their original start point
- Once the repetitions are completed, lower the hips and torso to the floor to bring the body to rest

Technical tips
- Keep the ankles, knees, hips, spine and shoulders in good alignment and as stable as possible during the plank hold. The head should also be in line with the eyes looking directly at the ground. Avoid looking up and extending the neck
- As each hand is lifted off the ground in turn to walk forward, the gravitational pull on the side of the body without arm support will create a rotational force that needs to be resisted and controlled by the core muscles to maintain good spinal alignment
- The greater the distance walked forward by the hands the greater the pendulum effect and resulting exercise intensity. The distance walked may be used progressively based on client ability
- As the core muscles begin to fatigue the body will tend to revert to its dominant postural position where it feels strongest, which is often not optimal plank position. Avoid the pelvis tilting forwards and arching of the lower back. Avoid excessive mid-back curvature or the hips raised high out of alignment. Avoid pelvic rotation where one side of the body or one hip sags lower than the other
- Cease the exercise if good spinal position cannot be maintained

Exercise 30 Suspended plank with rotational reach

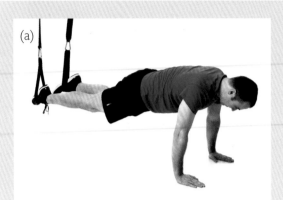
(a)

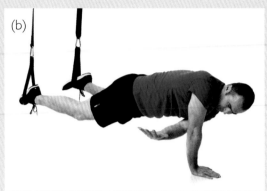
(b)

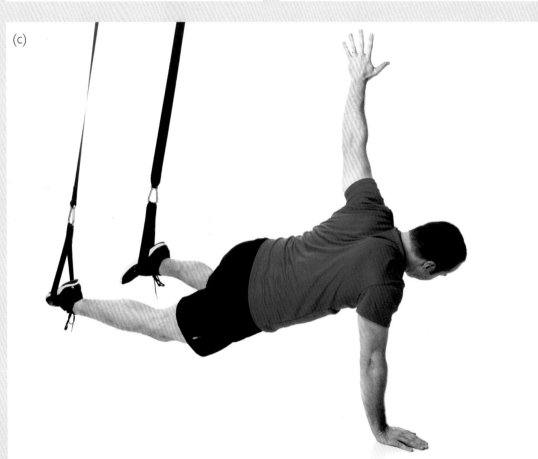
(c)

Target muscles: Abdominals, iliopsoas and obliques
Technique rating: 3
Intensity rating: 2
Challenge rating: 5

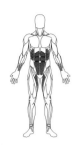

Set-up

Straps anchored high and set at long range. Foot loops attached

Positioning

Begin lying face down with feet set in the foot loops and elbows and forearms on the ground

Quick guide

- Lift the hips off the ground and push up off the elbows on to the hands with elbows locked out. Keep hips in alignment with the shoulders and feet in the loops and there is good spinal position
- Draw the feet apart and hold in a wider position to help control the rotational forces
- While maintaining good hip alignment lift one hand off the ground and reach under and across the body to the opposite side drawing the body into a rotated position
- Draw the hand back from under the body and reach outwards and above the body with the same hand rotating the body in the opposite direction
- Return the hand to the ground, change hands and repeat the same two reaches with the other arm
- Once the repetitions are completed, lower the hips and torso to the floor to bring the body to rest

Technical tips

- Keep the ankles, knees, hips, spine and shoulders in good alignment and relatively stable during the rotational reaches. The head should follow the hand with eyes looking at the hand as it reaches under and over the body
- As each hand is lifted off the ground in turn to perform the rotational reaches, gravitational pull on the side of the body without arm support will create a downward rotational force that needs to be resisted and controlled by the core muscles to maintain good spinal alignment. Rotation of the spine is necessary in the performance of the exercise, but too much extension of the spine should be avoided
- As the core muscles begin to fatigue the body will tend to revert to its dominant postural position where it feels strongest, which is often not optimal plank position. Avoid the pelvis tilting forwards and arching of the lower back. Avoid excessive mid-back curvature or the hips raised high out of alignment. Avoid pelvic rotation where one side of the body or one hip sags lower than the other
- Cease the exercise if good spinal position cannot be maintained

Exercise 31 Suspended walking jackknife

(a)

(b)

(c)

(d)

Target muscles:
  Abdominals, iliopsoas
  and deltoids
Technique rating: 3
Intensity rating: 3
Challenge rating: 6

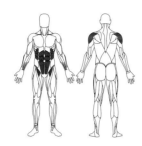

Set-up

Straps anchored high and set at long range. Foot loops attached

Positioning

Begin lying face down with feet set in the foot loops and elbows and forearms on the ground

Quick guide

• Lift the hips off the ground, push up on to the hands and hold the body in good alignment between the hands on the ground and feet suspended in the loops
• Walk forwards on the hands a few steps drawing the straps forward while maintaining good hip and back alignment
• Bend the hips and knees drawing the legs under the body up towards the chest
• Try to keep the pelvis down by pulling the knees underneath the body. Some upward motion will occur as the straps will arc forward and upwards around the anchor point drawing the body upwards
• Control the return movement, extending the hips and knees and walk back on the hands to the original position

Technical tips

• The walking jackknife requires a high degree of stabilisation through the torso and shoulders while simultaneously controlling movement at the legs and keeping strong through the shoulders and arms
• As the straps are moving around a fixed anchor point they will arc upwards lifting the feet in the loops as the knees are drawn under the body. This upward motion in the walking jackknife will likely be too great to compensate for and will lift the pelvis and back upwards to some degree
• Despite the upward arcing motion the intention is still to draw the knees under the body until the hips are beyond 90 degrees of flexion, ideally towards 120 degrees of flexion or thereabouts
• The greater the distance walked forward by the hands the greater the pendulum effect and resulting exercise intensity. The distance walked may be used progressively based on client ability

Exercise 32 Suspended jackknife twist

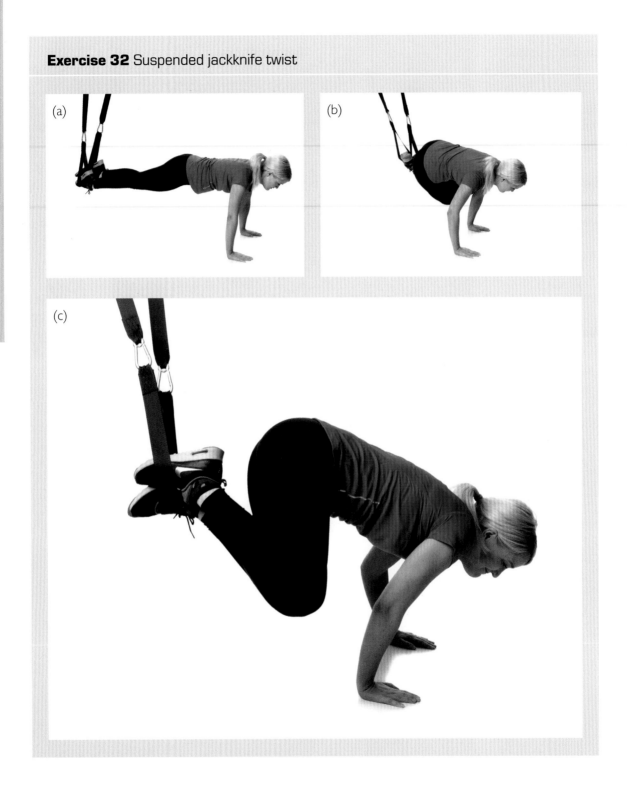

(a)

(b)

(c)

Target muscles:
Abdominals, iliopsoas, deltoids and obliques

Technique rating: 3

Intensity rating: 3

Challenge rating: 6

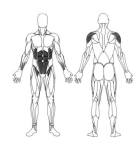

Set-up
Straps anchored high and set at long range. Foot loops attached

Positioning
Begin lying face down with feet set in the foot loops and elbows and forearms on the ground

Quick guide
- Lift the hips off the ground, push up on to the hands and hold the body in good alignment between the hands on the ground and feet suspended in the loops
- Bend the hips and knees drawing the legs under the body up towards the chest
- As the hips pass a 90-degree bend the knees being kept together should be drawn further forwards and outwards to one side of the body causing the torso to twist
- Keep the pelvis at a similar height as the shoulders throughout the whole movement
- Control the return movement, extending the hips and knees. Repeat the next repetition pulling the knees forwards and out towards the opposite side

Technical tips
- The jackknife twist requires a high degree of stabilisation through the torso and at the shoulder complex while simultaneously controlling movement at the legs
- As the straps are moving around a fixed anchor point they will arc upwards slightly lifting the feet in the loops as the knees are drawn under the body
- It is desirable to be able to draw the knees forwards until the hips are beyond 90 degrees of flexion, ideally towards 120 degrees of flexion or thereabouts
- Drawing the knees out to the sides will bring about spinal rotation and involve the oblique muscles as they control the movement and resist gravity. Approximately 30–40 degrees of rotation would be desirable each way

Exercise 33 Suspended jackknife pike

(a)

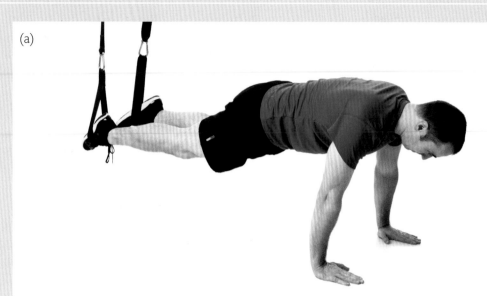

(b)

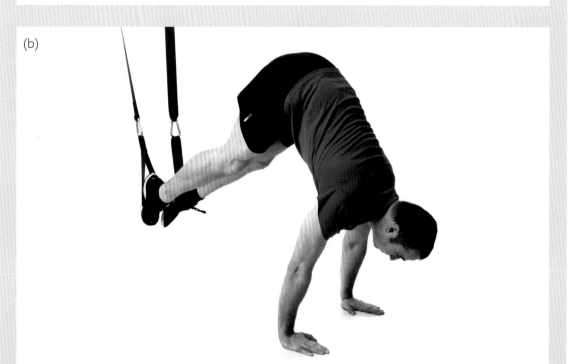

Target muscles:
Abdominals, iliopsoas
and deltoids
Technique rating: 3
Intensity rating: 3
Challenge rating: 6

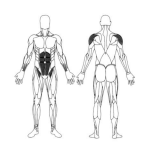

Set-up

Straps anchored high and set at long range. Foot loops attached

Positioning

Begin lying face down with feet set in the foot loops and elbows and forearms on the ground

Quick guide

- Lift the hips off the ground, push up on to the hands and hold the body in good alignment between the hands on the ground and feet suspended in the loops
- Bend the hips only keeping the knees straight and draw the hips upwards so that the body forms an inverted V position
- The body will be above the hands and shoulders at the top of the movement so that the shoulders will need to stabilise and hold position in a locked out inverted press
- Control the return movement as the hips lower down back into alignment and parallel with the ground once again

Technical tips

- The jackknife pike requires a high degree of strength through the torso and more particularly at the shoulder complex as the load on the shoulders will increase the more the hips bend and rise above the rest of the body
- The straps will be drawn forward during hip flexion and will create a pendulum effect that will pull against the legs and increase resistance for the iliopsoas and abdominals to control
- As the straps are moving around a fixed anchor point they will arc upwards slightly lifting the feet in the loops as the pike position is reached. This small upward motion will further shift centre of gravity over the shoulders

Exercise 34 Reverse cycling plank

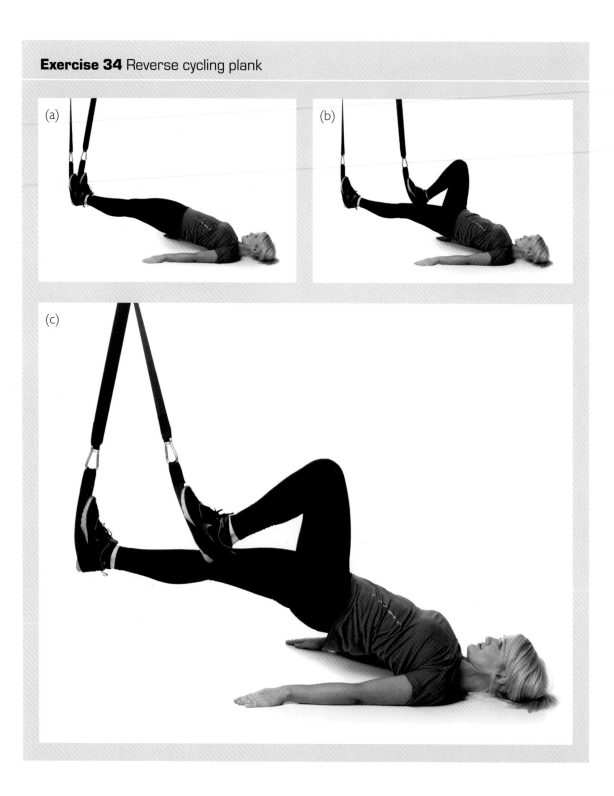

(a)

(b)

(c)

Target muscles: Hamstrings, gluteals and erector spinae

Technique rating: 2

Intensity rating: 3

Challenge rating: 5

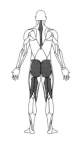

Set-up

Straps anchored high and set at long range. Foot loops attached

Positioning

Begin lying down on your back with heels set in the foot loops, shoulder blades on the ground and the hips lifted into alignment with feet and shoulders

Quick guide

- Bend the hip and knee of the left leg, drawing the foot and strap forwards until the foot is close to the buttocks
- While returning the left leg under control begin the movement of the right foot up towards the buttocks by bending the hip and knee on the right leg
- Repeat these movements in a cycling action
- Keep the pelvis raised off the ground throughout to maintain alignment with the straight leg position and the shoulders on the ground

Technical tips

- During this exercise the hips are bending and lengthening one end of the hamstrings while the knees are simultaneously bending which is shortening the other end of the hamstrings. It is the contraction of the hamstrings closer to the knees that resists the downward pull of gravity and generates the load that is experienced during the exercise
- Holding the pelvis in alignment is easy to focus on when the hips are held in a static extended position. The cycling leg action means that one or both hips are moving in and out of flexion at any one time and it is easy to lose focus on body alignment and to let the pelvis and low back drop downwards towards the ground. It may be helpful to hold hands on the ground directly under the mid-back so that if it drops and contacts the back of the hands at any point it will serve as an early warning that the body is losing alignment and the pelvis can be raised again

Exercise 35 Reverse plank with hamstring drags

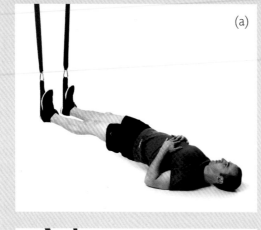

(a)

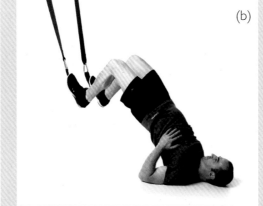

(b)

Positioning

Begin lying down on your back with heels set in the foot loops, shoulder blades on the ground and the hips lifted into alignment with feet and shoulders

Quick guide

- Bend the knees only drawing the foot and strap forwards until the knees are at right angles
- Keep the hips raised in a fixed extended position through the exercise
- Hands and arms should ideally be placed across the chest, but if balance is a challenge they can be placed either side on the ground
- Pull into the positive phase of motion quickly and control the negative phase of motion more slowly back to the start position

Technical tips

- The body remains fixed from the hips to the shoulders in a reverse plank position and the only movement in this exercise comes from the flexion and extension of the knees
- The combination of increased body weight load and increased pendulum effect during the flexing of the knees creates a very intense resistance that is targeted primarily in the hamstring group

Target muscles: Hamstrings, gluteals and erector spinae
Technique rating: 2
Intensity rating: 4
Challenge rating: 6

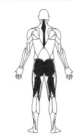

Set-up

Straps anchored high and set at long range. Foot loops attached

SUSPEND AND STRETCH

7

Post-exercise flexibility is an important aspect in any training programme. It has been known for many years that during an acute bout of exercise muscle tissue will shorten in length and become tighter than in the pre-exercise state. While this is a temporary state which is usually rectified with rest over a couple of days, the restoration of muscle tissue to pre-exercise lengths can be achieved quicker by including a stretching and flexibility programme.

Post-exercise stretching serves a very different purpose to pre-exercise mobility work – but this is often not understood. You may know people who do no stretching at all or if they do stretch it would only be one set of stretches, either before or after, but not both. However, the job is only half done. Whereas pre-exercise mobility is focused on warming up, activating and lengthening previously rested muscle tissue in readiness for exercise, post-exercise stretches restore length in muscle tissue that has shortened as a result of applied exercise, cools the muscle down, eases out feelings of tension and helps shift the body away from stress response, as is the case during exercise, towards a more relaxed state that will aid exercise recovery.

Let's delve a bit deeper into the anatomy and physiology. Muscle tissue has a dense network of small blood vessels called capillaries that help to ensure every part of the muscle is supplied with blood and oxygen, which is used to produce energy at a cellular level. The more effectively blood can be supplied to the muscle, the more oxygen is available for aerobic energy production. Increasing heart rate and consistent movement helps to dilate the blood vessels and capillaries enabling blood to flow more effectively into the working muscles. Applying motionless, end-of-range positions to stretch the muscles, or static stretches, is clearly not effective at improving and maintaining blood supply to the muscles. However, in the cool-down period at the end of an exercise session, maintaining high-volume blood supply to the muscles is no longer important and doing some static stretches is more appropriate.

Muscles also have a complex nervous system to control and regulate the range of contraction, the force of contraction and the speed at which a contraction occurs. One of the structures that help to regulate this is a microscopic control centre called the muscle spindle. Muscle spindles are connected to the individual muscle fibres and provide a sensitive and rapid response mechanism for the nervous system to regulate muscle contraction. Muscle spindles are activated by changes in the length of a muscle and by the speed at which muscle tissue changes length. The greater the length of the muscle and the faster the muscle changes length the more the muscle spindle stimulates neural signals and vice versa. Think of it a bit like an old fashioned church bell. The faster and greater distance the rope is pulled, the louder and more often the bell will ring. The muscle spindle is like a neurological bell that rings to notify the central nervous system that a response is required. The outcome of the nervous stimulus that the spindle creates is to cause a contraction within the same muscle tissue. Therefore, the greater level of muscle spindle activation the greater the level of resulting muscle contraction that will occur. This knowledge of muscle spindle mechanics has greatly influenced the way in which flexibility work is applied.

Over the years warm-up work has moved away from the inclusion of static stretches and now the recommendations are to apply dynamic, mobility work instead. This is engaging in large rhythmical movements, beginning slowly with shorter range, then progressing the range and speed of movement. Applying movement in this way helps to activate the muscle spindles in preparation for the exercise that is to follow. Dynamic mobility provides an important stimulus for improving muscular contraction. This chapter will provide a broad range of mobility exercises that will help improve muscle activation and function as part of a warm-up. This activating of muscle spindles has been shown to decrease injury risk more effectively than static stretching, in fact in some scientific studies static stretching before exercise has been shown to increase injury risk.

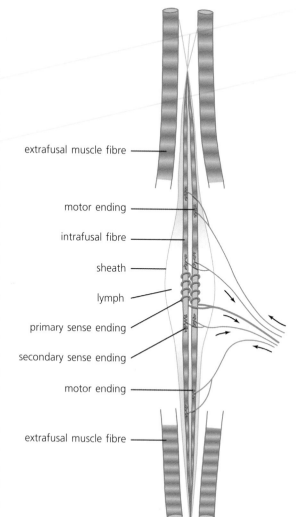

extrafusal muscle fibre

motor ending

intrafusal fibre

sheath

lymph

primary sense ending

secondary sense ending

motor ending

extrafusal muscle fibre

Figure 7.1 Diagram of a muscle spindle

During the initial eight to ten seconds of a static stretch the increased range of motion that has been created by moving a muscle or group of muscles into a stretch position pulls the muscle spindles apart, stimulating muscular contraction. This phenomenon is known as the stretch reflex. Muscle spindle activation is what creates the pulling sensation during the first few seconds of positioning a body part into a stretch position. However, during the initial ten seconds or so of stretch the muscle is not lengthening, but undergoing contraction and no improvement in muscle length occurs. This is the reason why typical stretching guidelines indicate that static stretching should be held for 20 to 30 seconds. When a static stretch position is held for this longer duration of time the stretch reflex response adapts. Muscle spindle activity diminishes after a short period of being held motionless in an elongated position. A reduction in spindle activity allows muscle contraction to ease off and even cease after approximately 15 to 20 seconds of holding a static stretch position. Once the contraction switches off the muscle is able to gradually lengthen and benefit from the stretch. In essence, the spindles adapt to the new muscle length and they are in a way recalibrated to the new lengthened position. Understanding this important aspect of body physiology provides two vital principles in relation to static stretching:

- Static stretching must be held long enough for spindle activity to adapt and switch off or increased muscle length will not be achieved
- Proper static stretching held long enough to lengthen muscle tissue resets the stretch reflex and reduces muscle responsiveness to changes in muscle length

These two principles make it clear that static stretching is not effective for a warm-up − in fact it's counterproductive as it reduces muscle responsiveness to the rapid changes of length that will occur during exercise. It also teaches that after an exercise session has been completed static stretching is completely appropriate and reasonably effective at restoring muscle tissue length providing it is applied properly over time and not

rushed, in other words holding for a full 20 to 30 seconds for each stretch.. However, some chronically tight muscles may be a little more stubborn and may require longer than the guideline 20 to 30 seconds before the stretch reflex diminishes and allows the tissues to lengthen. Pay close attention during the stretching of very tight muscles and be aware of the initiation of the stretch reflex and wait patiently until the muscle is felt to ease off and relax − then you know that a change in muscle length has occurred as a result of applying a static stretch.

If you have really tight muscles you can apply two or three phases of static stretch to really make improvement in the resting muscle length. This can be carried out as follows:

- Hold a stretch position for approximately 20 to 30 seconds or until the stretch reflex subsides and a small increase in muscle length is experienced
- Move further into the stretch position increasing the target muscle's length until the stretch reflex is activated again
- Hold the new position for approximately 20 to 30 seconds or until the stretch reflex subsides and a small increase in muscle length is experienced
- Repeat one more time if needed

So, dynamic mobility should be part of your warm-up, and static stretches are an effective part of the cool-down. The rest of this chapter will outline static stretches you can use as part of your cool-down programme. While the majority of muscles can be stretched without any equipment, the use of suspended fitness straps can be a helpful addition in providing effective static stretching.

Muscle stretch Calf complex

(a)

(b)

(c)

(d)

(e)

(f)

Set-up

Straps anchored high and set at short range. Handles attached

Quick guide

- Face away from the anchor point and pass straps under the armpits and grip the handles close to the sides of the chest, leaning forward to place tension through the straps
- Take up a large split stance with the back knee kept straight, heel on the ground and body weight supported by the front leg and the straps
- Lunge into the forward leg creating a sharper angle at the rear ankle and stimulating a stretch in the calf complex; hold until the stretch reflex subsides
- Vary the direction of the lunge for different stretching angles, both medially and laterally across the posterior leg calf complex

Non-suspended alternative

- Take up a large split stance with the back knee kept straight, heel on the ground and body weight supported by the front leg with the arms leaning against an object such as a wall
- Lunge into the forward leg creating a sharper angle at the rear ankle and stimulating a stretch in the calf complex, hold until the stretch reflex subsides
- Vary the direction of the lunge for different stretching angles, both medially and laterally across the posterior leg calf complex

Muscle stretch Hamstrings

(a)

(b)

(c)

(d)

(e)

(f)

Set-up

Straps anchored high and set at short range. Handles attached

Quick guide

- Face towards the anchor point and grip the handles, leaning back to place tension through the straps
- Take up a split stance with body weight on the bent back leg and the front leg knee kept straight with the heel on the ground and the toe in the air
- Inch the feet backward across the floor away from the handles and flex forward at the hips to bring the front leg hamstring into a lengthened position while still maintaining tension through the straps at all times
- Hold until the stretch reflex subsides
- Rotate the foot outwards to target the inner hamstrings (semimembranosus and semitendinosus) and hold until the stretch reflex subsides then repeat again with the foot rotated inwards to target the outer hamstrings (biceps femoris)

Non-suspended alternative

- Kneel down on one knee with the other leg placed straight out in front of the body without locking the knee joint, keeping the heel on the ground and the toe in the air
- Draw the hips back slightly and reach forwards towards the front foot to initiate the stretch
- Hold until the stretch reflex subsides
- Rotate the foot outwards to target the inner hamstrings (semimembranosus and semitendinosus) and hold until the stretch reflex subsides then repeat again with the foot rotated inwards to target the outer hamstrings (biceps femoris)

Muscle stretch Adductors

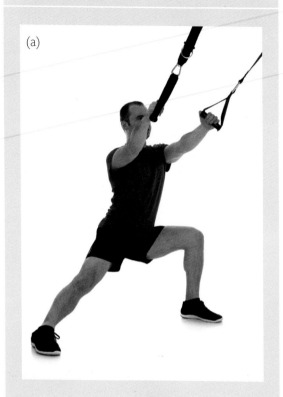

(a)

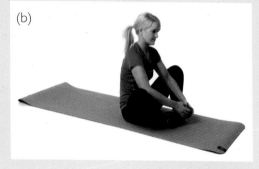

(b)

Set-up
Straps anchored high and set at short range. Handles attached

Quick guide
- Face towards the anchor point and grip the handles, leaning back to place tension through the straps
- Take a wide lateral lunge stance with body weight on the outer bent leg with the inside leg knee kept straight and the sole of the foot on the ground
- Drop deeper into the lateral lunge to stretch the trail leg adductor while still maintaining tension through the straps at all times to help support body weight
- Hold until the stretch reflex within the adductor subsides

Non-suspended alternative
- Sit on the ground with the soles of the feet together and the knees allowed to fall out wide
- Draw the feet in close to the pelvis with the hands and use the elbows to press against the legs pushing the knees down towards the ground to initiate the stretch
- Hold until the stretch reflex within the adductors subside

Muscle stretch Gluteals

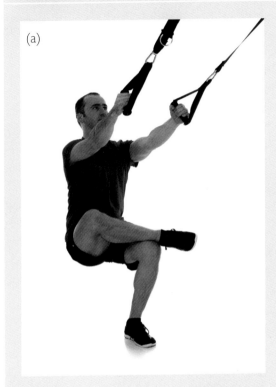

(a)

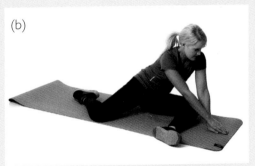

(b)

Set-up
Straps anchored high and set at short range. Handles attached

Quick guide
- Face towards the anchor point and grip the handles, leaning back to place tension through the straps
- Stand on one leg and cross the other foot onto the knee of the stance leg
- Drop down into a single-leg squat position supporting body weight with the straps
- Allow the knee of the crossed leg to drop out wide
- Drive the hips back and down to feel the stretch reflex initiate in the gluteals
- Hold until the stretch reflex within the gluteals subsides

Non-suspended alternative
- Sit on the ground with one leg in front of the body with the outside of the knee on the ground and joint at a right angle
- The other leg is held out to the side with the inside of the knee against the ground and the joint at a right angle
- Reach directly in front of the body with hands on the ground to feel the stretch reflex initiate in the gluteals
- Hold until the stretch reflex within the gluteals subsides

Muscle stretch Iliopsoas or hip flexors

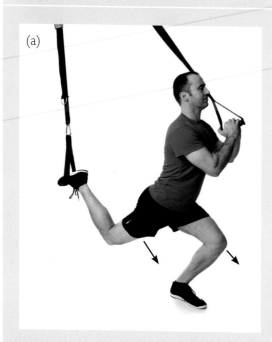

(a)

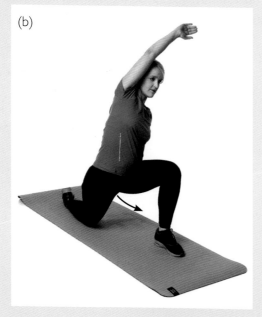

(b)

Set-up

Straps anchored high and set at long range. One foot loop and one handle attached

Quick guide

- Face away from the anchor point and place one foot into the long foot loop, hold the other handle with the strap running over the shoulder
- Inch forward along the ground so that the leg in the loop is drawn back behind the body
- Drop into a lunge position and push the hips forward stretching the rear leg iliopsoas
- Maintain tension through both straps to help keep balanced
- Hold until the stretch reflex within the iliopsoas subsides

Non-suspended alternative

- Kneel down on one knee in a split-lunge position and push the hips forward, initiating a stretch within the rear leg iliopsoas
- Reach the same side arm as the stretching leg up overhead and across to the opposite side of the body while maintaining the forward hip stretch position
- Hold until the stretch reflex within the iliopsoas subsides

Muscle stretch Abdominals

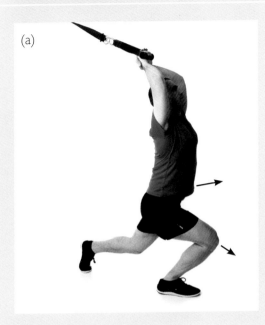

(a)

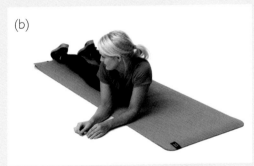

(b)

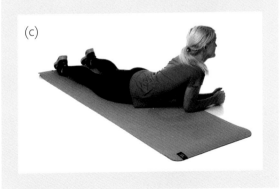

(c)

Set-up
Straps anchored high and set at short range. Handles attached

Quick guide
- Face away from the anchor point and grip the handles overhead, leaning forward to place some gentle tension through the straps
- Take a small split stance and inch forward drawing the arms further behind and allowing the spine to extend. Care should be taken not to cause any pain or discomfort in the lower back
- The hips should remain in flexion so as not to target and stretch the iliopsoas
- Keeping the arms high, reach over to the side with the forward leg, laterally flexing the spine to initiate a stretch reflex across one side of the abdominals
- Hold the position until the stretch reflex within the abdominals subsides then repeat by switching legs and reaching to the opposite side

Non-suspended alternative
- Lie face down then push up on to the elbows and look upwards elongating the abdominals
- If the stretch is not sufficient then push up on to the hands and ensure the hips remain in contact with the ground
- Walk the elbows or hands round to one side of the body and hold to stretch the opposite side of the abdominals
- Hold until the stretch reflex within the abdominals subsides then repeat by switching hands over to the opposite side

Muscle stretch Erector spinae

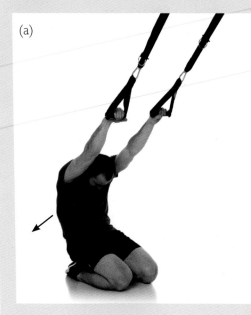

(a)

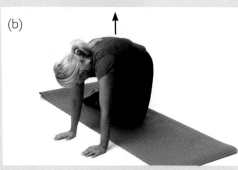

(b)

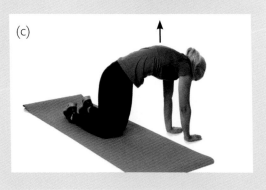

(c)

Set-up
Straps anchored high and set at medium range. Handles attached

Quick guide
- Face towards the anchor point and kneel down gripping both handles, inching back to place tension through the straps
- Kneel right down to bring the hips on top of the feet and arch the back, pushing it behind the body while simultaneously drawing the chin into the chest
- Hold until the stretch reflex within the erector spinae subsides

Non-suspended alternative
- Begin kneeling on all fours in a box position
- Arch the back and push the middle of the back upwards towards the ceiling and tuck the chin down close to the chest
- Walk the hands round to one side keeping the same arched back position to feel the stretch down one side erector spinae
- Hold until the stretch reflex within the erector spinae subsides then walk hands to the other side and repeat

Muscle stretch Latissimus dorsi

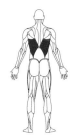

Set-up
Straps anchored high and set at short range. Handles attached

Quick guide
- Face 45 degrees to one side of the anchor point and grip a single handle
- Take a wide stance simultaneously reaching the arm holding the handle overhead back towards the anchor point
- Inch away until the strap has some mild tension then drop into a wide lateral lunge away from the anchor point to pull the arm further across and initiate the stretch reflex
- Hold until the stretch reflex within the latissimus dorsi subsides

Non-suspended alternative
- Kneel down on to all fours in a box position
- Reach one arm at full length in front of the body with the outer edge of the hand against the ground with the thumb pointing up
- Draw the extended arm across to the opposite side and drop the shoulder down towards the ground to initiate the stretch
- Hold until the stretch reflex within the latissimus dorsi subsides then repeat on the opposite side

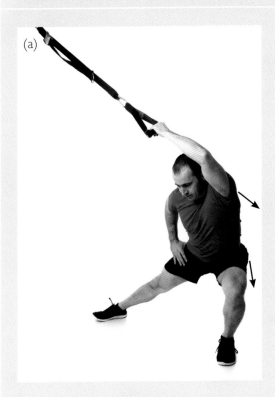

(a)

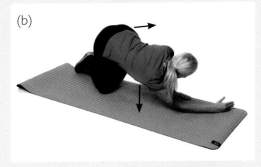

(b)

Muscle stretch Mid-trapezius and rhomboids

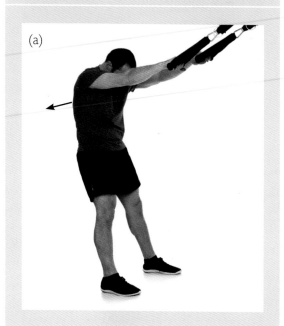

(a)

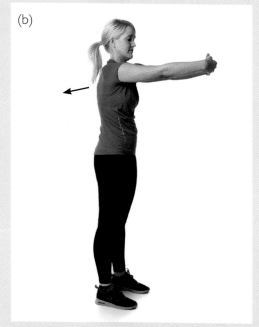

(b)

Set-up
Straps anchored high and set at short range. Handles attached

Quick guide
- Face towards the anchor point and grip both handles, leaning back to place gentle tension through the straps
- Take a split stance to help control the tension placed through the muscles and ensure it does not continually increase
- Lean back more firmly allowing the shoulders to round forward and drop the chin into the chest, stretching the mid-trapezius and rhomboid muscles
- Hold until the stretch reflex within the target muscles subsides

Non-suspended alternative
- Reach both arms in front of the body at shoulder height with the hands clasped together
- Push the elbows outwards and the shoulders forward and drop the chin into the chest stretching the mid-trapezius and rhomboid muscles
- Hold until the stretch reflex within the target muscles subsides

Muscle stretch Pectorals

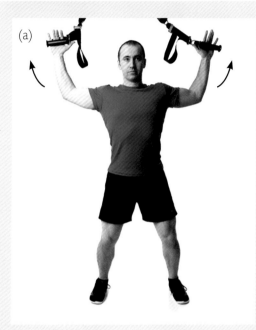

(a)

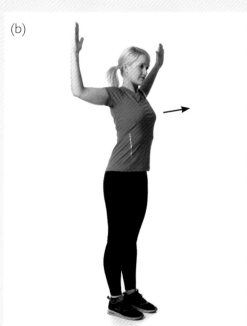

(b)

Set-up
Straps anchored high and set at short range. Handles attached

Quick guide
- Face away from the anchor point and grip the handles high with arms raised overhead and elbows at right angles on either side
- Take a split stance and inch forward to place gentle tension through the straps
- Drop into a partial forward lunge to draw the raised arms against the straps so they move behind the body initiating a stretch reflex within the pectorals
- Hold position until the stretch reflex within the target muscles subsides then repeat on the other arm

Non-suspended alternative
- Place the arm high against an object such as a wall with the elbow at a right angle and the forearm in full contact
- Turn the body away from the raised arm and look back over the opposite shoulder to initiate a stretch reflex within the pectorals
- Hold position until the stretch reflex within the target muscle subsides then repeat on the other arm

Muscle stretch Posterior deltoids

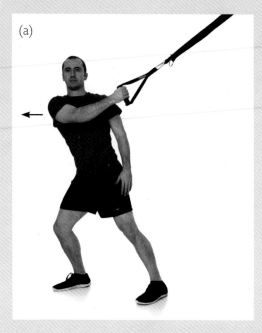

(a)

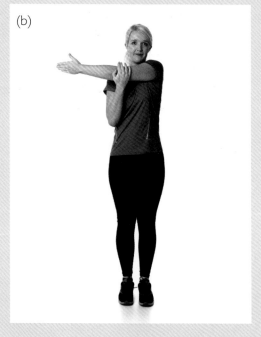

(b)

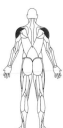

Set-up
Straps anchored high and set at short range. Handles attached

Quick guide
- Face away at 90 degrees to the anchor point reaching across the body to grip a single handle at shoulder height
- Take a wide stance and partially lunge on to the outer leg to increase the tension in the straps and pull the arm tight across the body initiating a stretch across the posterior shoulder
- Hold until the stretch reflex within the posterior deltoid subsides

Non-suspended alternative
- Bring one arm across the body to the opposite side at shoulder height
- Using the free hand grab the elbow of the arm to be stretched and pull it in towards the body to initiate a stretch reflex
- Hold until the stretch reflex within the posterior deltoid subsides then repeat on the other side

Muscle stretch Biceps brachii

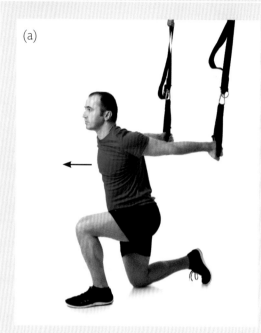

(a)

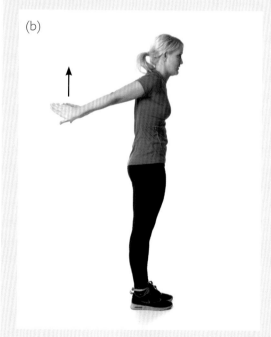

(b)

Set-up
Straps anchored high and set at short range. Handles attached

Quick guide
- Face away from the anchor point and grip the handles behind the body at around hip height, stepping forward to place some tension through the straps
- Kneel down on to the knees and inch forward so the arms are raised directly behind the body
- If a stretch is still not felt then drop into a low kneeling position by sitting on the feet and push the chest forwards and up
- Hold until the stretch reflex within the biceps subsides

Non-suspended alternative
- Place one arm straight behind the body so that the knuckles of the hand are in contact with a wall at approximately shoulder height and the thumb is pointing downwards
- Keeping the hand in position lower the body downwards to initiate a stretch in the biceps
- Hold until the stretch reflex within the biceps subsides and repeat on the other arm

Muscle stretch Triceps brachii

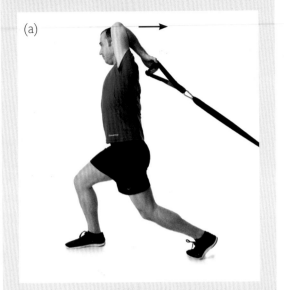

(a)

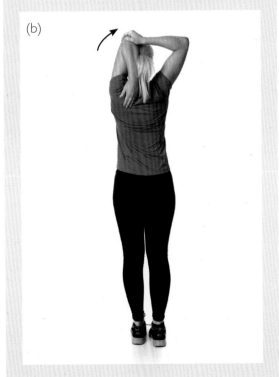

(b)

Set-up

Single straps anchored very low down and set at medium range. Handle attached.

Quick guide

- Face away from the anchor point in a split stance and drop into a partial lunge to grip the handle behind the head with elbow flexed as much as possible
- Handle should be kept close to the shoulder and scapula at all times
- Rise up out of the partial lunge to increase the tension in the straps and to create a downward pull on the handle creating a stretch in the triceps
- Hold until the stretch reflex within the triceps subsides then lower down into a partial lunge to release the position and switch hands to repeat on the opposite side

Non-suspended alternative

- Raise one arm up overhead and bend the elbow bringing the hand in behind the shoulder tight to the shoulder blade
- Using the other arm reach up and grab the elbow that is pointing upwards
- Gently pull the elbow across as though trying to bring it behind the head
- Keep the hand on the stretching side tight the shoulder blade at all times
- Hold until the stretch reflex within the triceps subsides then repeat on the other arm

PROGRAMME DESIGN 8

Now that we've covered the separate mobilisations, exercises and stretches that comprise a typical exercise programme, these need drawing together to produce a flowing and effective workout and also to help create a long-term exercise programme.

Sometimes in life we categorise individuals into various groups to help us understand where we stand, to provide identity and the ability to relate to other like-minded people. One very simplistic category breakdown is to split people into planners and doers. It is likely that those who relate to being 'doers' may find the idea of creating a long-term exercise plan unnecessary and maybe even a little annoying as it will slow down the application of the training they are so keen to get started with and delay the benefits and results they are seeking. The individuals who relate to being 'planners' will be in their element here and will enjoy the process of learning how to develop an exercise programme and how to track physical progress and plan the achievement of their fitness objectives. They will see the plan as an integral part of reaching their goals.

There is something to be learnt from both types of people. The 'doers' need to recognise that rushing into a new fitness programme without planning carefully in advance can lead to errors being made and less effective training being carried out,

ultimately slowing the rate at which their fitness goals are reached. Ironically, the rapid attainment of their goals may well be the reason these types of people tend to rush into an exercise programme in the first place. The 'planners' may struggle to adhere to a well thought-out exercise programme even if is laid out in front of them as their own internal motivations may run out of steam too early to see the benefits their carefully devised plan could have delivered.

The driving motivation to get busy 'doing' tends to be inconsistent and wanes from time to time. The 'doers' may not need to master every aspect and variable of fitness planning, but stick with this chapter and learn the important keys that will ensure your plans, even if fairly brief, will serve you well and help you achieve your objectives in an efficient manner. The 'planners' need to be motivated enough to get going a little bit sooner, rather than later, and find a deeper-rooted motivation that will serve them well so that they will adhere to an exercise programme long enough to reap the benefits and achieve their objectives. Effective programme design combined with determined, sustained action in a logical, progressive manner will help to reach your desired training objectives quicker with fewer mistakes along the way.

RECORD-KEEPING

An essential part of creating a plan is to write it down. If you have mapped out a plan in your mind, during exercise, you may forget one or two components, whereas having a plan in front of you tells you exactly what exercise to do and in what order.

An exercise plan should begin with a training overview that identifies the key objectives and breaks the journey down into a few smaller phases. Each smaller phase should also have a goal that should be reached when each shorter phase is completed.

WARM UP				
Exercise	Speed/ rpm	Incline / Level	Duration	Notes
CV:				
Dynamic mobility:				

MAIN SESSION				TRAINING RECORD				
Exercise	Sets/ reps	Rest	Notes	Date:	Date:	Date:	Date:	Date:

COOL DOWN				
Exercise	Speed/ rpm	Incline/ Level	Duration	Notes
CV:				
Static stretches:				

Figure 8.1 Blank programme template

It is much easier to create an exercise programme by planning in smaller chunks than it is to create a whole, detailed master plan in one go.

For example, if a long-term goal, such as a 20% increase in physical performance, is set to be achieved in four months' time, this could be broken down into four one-month segments with shorter monthly goals. Each month is planned one at a time, rather than planning a detailed four-month period. The shorter month-long plans should have small adjustments from week to week that help progress the training within that time period. The exercise programming for months two to four would build upon the training completed in the first month in a structured process that leads to the primary objective.

The overall objective and the smaller goals should be recorded and written down. Weekly training plans should also be recorded and the successful completion of each element of a workout noted, along with a space for identifying small adjustments that were made from session to session. For example, a suspended chest press exercise may have been planned to perform 3 sets of 15 repetitions, but during the actual workout they were only able to complete 12 repetitions in the final set. This alteration to the plan should be recorded on the training record so that actual achievement is clearly visible as well as the intended plan. This is helpful information that will contribute to more accurate planning in the subsequent weeks. Figure 8.1 provides an example of a training record that could be used for planning and recording each workout.

ACUTE TRAINING VARIABLES

Good programme design should always build a progressive series of exercises upon the foundations laid down by the previous training phases. The ability to progress a training programme is dependent upon the management of the different acute or short term training variables. Each variable can play an important part in progressing or regressing the difficulty or purpose of a workout depending on each individual's needs. Each acute variable warrants a brief explanation of how it can impact upon a training session.

- **Set** – a series of exercise repetitions that are performed in a successive block. The number of sets to be performed is dependent on the training objective and an individual's current ability. More sets of a given exercise usually means greater training volume and more work performed by the targeted muscles, which in turn increases the training stimulus to adapt and develop. The number of sets for a given exercise normally ranges between 2 and 5 depending on the objective and ability of the exerciser.
- **Repetition** – the individual movements that make up one complete cycle of an exercise, such as the flexion and extension of the elbow that comprise a bicep curl. The number of repetitions performed within a given set will depend upon the training objective and an individual's current ability. Repetitions typically range from as low as 6 to as high as 20 in a single set. Lower down the scale usually requires a greater load and focuses on building strength and size of muscle. Higher up the scale requires a lesser load and focuses on muscular endurance and increasing muscle tone.
- **Rest period** – refers to the amount of time between sets of exercise. The amount of rest will depend upon the difficulty of the exercise and the number of repetitions performed. A lower

number of repetitions usually corresponds to a higher load being lifted and a greater degree of effort, which will then require a longer rest period. Enduring through a higher number of repetitions usually corresponds to a lighter load and a reduced level of total effort which then dictates a shorter rest period. Typically rest between sets ranges from 30 seconds for light, endurance work up to as long as 3 or 4 minutes in some cases for power and explosive exercises.

- **Angle of loading** – relates to the degree of resistance felt by the exerciser as a result of changing body angle to increase or decrease the percentage of body weight lifted during a suspended exercise (see chapter 4). Unlike using an external resistance, such as dumbbells or kettle bells, selecting the correct load in suspended fitness training requires a little more guess work as it is related to the angle of the body in relation to the contact point with the ground. A sharper angle means a greater load is being lifted.

- **Repetition speed** – refers to the rate at which a single repetition is performed and ranges from slow and controlled to fast and explosive. Both extremes increase the difficulty of the exercise. Slow repetitions increase the time that a muscle is kept under tension to perform a complete set and greater energy is expended. Faster, explosive repetitions require more effort to rapidly overcome gravity with each quick repetition. The time under tension during rapid movement is shorter, but the increased acceleration and deceleration of each repetition significantly raises the difficulty. In general a moderate repetition speed tends to be the easiest pace to work at and the one that most people feel comfortable with.

- **Number of exercises** – refers to how many exercises comprise a full workout. The number of exercises generally increases the volume of work to be performed in a single physical training session and increases the amount of total effort expended during a workout.

- **Exercise order** – the order that each exercise is to be performed in a workout can have an effect on the difficulty of the subsequent exercises. This will depend upon the muscles involved and the movement targeted. For example, if a full set of suspended chest press is followed by a suspended walking plank the quality of the second exercise may be negatively affected as the chest and shoulders will likely already be fatigued, making effective execution of the plank much harder. Even though the plank targets the core muscles, the fatigued chest and shoulder muscles are still involved to stabilise the body and perform the walking motions. This could be an unwanted side effect of poor planning. Alternatively it could be applied intentionally to create greater overload for these specific muscles. The rules to help effectively order exercises within a programme will be discussed shortly.

- **Training frequency** – the number of training sessions within a week. More sessions per week increases the overall training volume and increases the number of times that a stimulus to improve is applied. Increasing training frequency can, in the right circumstances, lead to quicker physical gains, but it can cause problems if it is not managed correctly. Exercising too often without adequate recovery can lead to over-training where physical development stagnates due to excessive stress and exercise-induced illness and injury risk increases.

- **Recovery** – refers to the time between training sessions where the body restores its energy reserves, repairs and rebuilds muscle tissue and other physical hardware. While the body will inherently strive to recover by itself between training it can be greatly supported by high-quality nutrition, minimising other stressors and ensuring enough good quality sleep is obtained. It is vital to understand that the body only really gets fitter and stronger during the recovery period. Exercise is an important stimulus to bring about physical development, but without effective recovery exercise alone will only serve to wear the body down and bring on fatigue and reduced performance. Determining a suitable recovery period will depend upon an individual's physical capacity as well as the intensity of the training performed. As a general rule deconditioned or older individuals may require longer recovery time between training sessions. Younger, fitter individuals usually recover quicker, though if there are other significant stressors, food quality is lacking and they are sleep-deprived, recovery may still be sluggish and more time will be required. An effective training programme will balance training frequency with the right amount of recovery time to match an individual's needs.

EXERCISE SELECTION

There are several criteria that need to be considered when selecting the exercises that will make up each workout. Identifying which movement patterns are required will help to target the correct sections of the exercise chapters, and then determining which muscle groups need to be worked may help to whittle down the choices even further. Each exercise listed in chapters 6 and 7 has the primary muscles that are worked identified in the description.

The next consideration is your own current physical ability. Each exercise is rated in terms of the difficulty of applying the correct technique and the level of intensity or effort required to perform the movements involved. These two guiding numbers combine to provide the overall exercise challenge rating which ranges from the easiest exercises rated at 1 or 2 through to the most difficult exercises rated at 7 or 8. You will also need to consider which phase of training is being focused on, such as joint stabilisation, muscular endurance, body-weight strength or speed power. Certain exercises will lend well to certain objectives and not to others. For example, a suspended squat jump can be an effective part of developing speed power, but is not really going to be as good at developing muscular endurance because the muscles will be working at very high intensity and they will fatigue quickly.

When selecting exercises, ensure there is enough variety to maintain your interest in the training programme. If every exercise selected is very basic they may be mastered too quickly, alternatively, if the exercises focus too much on the same movement pattern or body parts then the programme may quickly lose its appeal. Providing a range of exercises with variety and enjoyment can help to ensure the programme will have a bit more longevity and it will help maintain your motivation, making it more likely that you will stick to the programme.

To help provide a better idea regarding effective exercise selection it may be helpful to discuss a couple of theoretical examples. Imagine a beginner exerciser is seeking to lose weight and restore lost muscle tone particularly on their legs and abdominals. They require a selection of exercises that will help to deliver these two objectives. While there are many options that could work in this scenario, the following exercises could help to meet the individual's objectives:

1. Suspended squat (challenge 2 – see page 39)
2. Suspended lunge (challenge 4 – see page 46)
3. Suspended plank (challenge 3 – see page 52)
4. Suspended jackknife (challenge 4 – see page 55)

The targeted movement patterns and muscles involved meet the individual's needs and the exercises are not too complex or difficult in terms of their challenge rating. Please note that this is not a whole programme and would likely still require some upper body exercises to provide balance to the workout.

An experienced exerciser has just recently been introduced to suspended fitness training and is keen to use this form of exercise to help develop their power and explosiveness to assist with their sprint capacity. Again there could be several different ways to meet this goal. The following exercises offer one solution that will help to meet their needs:

1. Single-leg squats (challenge 4 – see page 41)
2. Suspended squat jumps (challenge 4 – see page 42)
3. Low to high straight-arm pull (challenge 5 – see page 75)
4. Hip thrust narrow row and reach (challenge 5 – see page 78)
5. Jumping sprint starts (challenge 6 – see page 102)
6. Hanging ice skater (challenge 7 – see page 98)
7. rotational reach (challenge 5 – see page 110)

These exercises provide a range of movement patterns that will aid in sprint work including explosive leg work, single-leg training, hip drives and arm drives. It also includes rotational core work as sprinting is heavily dependent upon effective rotation of the torso.

To have an effective programme it is important that the combination of exercises does not create so much challenge that the individual is worn out halfway through. The individual described above is also new to suspended fitness training so even though they are an advanced exerciser, they will need some more straight forward exercises that they should be able to master more quickly, hence a range of options across the challenge rating scale.

The key with regard to exercise selection is to consider and have suitable justification for why each exercise has been selected in relation to the fitness objectives being targeted. It is also wise to ensure that there is still room for exercise progression beyond just simply adapting the sets, repetitions and rest periods. Over time it is important to change and alter the exercises within the programme as this helps with enjoyment, varies the stimulus and can allow the challenge of the programme to gradually move upwards.

EXERCISE ORDER

Once the exercises have been selected it is important to organise them into an effective order to aid the flow and to ensure excess muscle fatigue does not become a problem midway through a workout. Many suspension exercises involve the whole body and it can be a little tricky to plan a routine strictly in line with the basic exercise order guidelines. However, most exercises will involve a primary muscle or group of muscles that the exercise emphasises. Understanding the primary muscles for each exercise can help you meet, or get close to meeting, the ordering guidelines. All the exercises listed in chapters 6 and 7 have the primary target muscles identified which will aid this process.

There are a few simple rules that can serve as your basis for ordering exercises successfully.

1. Complex movements and/or larger muscles targeted earlier in the session
2. Simpler movements and/or smaller muscles targeted later in the session
3. Seek to balance muscles and/or movements within an exercise session or across a training week
4. Specific core exercises targeted last in the session

EXERCISE COMPLEXITY

Performing complex exercises with a higher challenge rating, especially those with a high technique rating, can be very taxing on the nervous system and it is good to focus on these earlier in the workout when the body and brain are still fresh and attention to technique will be highest. It is more likely if they are left to the end that exercise technique will be less accurate due to fatigue built up from the earlier exercises and that will likely increase risk of injury. Simpler movements with reduced technical demand can be left to later in a workout as they carry less risk of going wrong or of being executed poorly.

MUSCLE SIZE

Larger muscles or muscle groups tend to have greater capacity to resist fatigue and to perform at higher levels. Smaller muscles usually fatigue sooner. In many compound or multi-joint exercises

both large and small muscle groups are involved simultaneously. For example, a suspended chest press targets both the large pectorals across the chest and the smaller triceps in the back of the upper arms, but the greater load is experienced by the pectorals. During a suspended triceps dip the same two muscle groups are involved, but in this case the triceps take the brunt of the load as the pectorals play a secondary stabilising role. The exercise order rules state that the chest press should be performed earlier than the triceps dip. The larger pectorals, being more fatigue resistant, will most likely still be able to stabilise the triceps dip even after a few sets of chest press have been performed. However, the triceps are smaller muscles and more prone to fatigue. It is very likely that if the dips were performed first the triceps would fail too early in the performance of the chest press exercise preventing sufficient work on the chest muscles.

MUSCULAR BALANCE

Muscular balance refers to ensuring that all body parts are trained to an appropriate and evenly matched volume and intensity. There are different ways in which this can be achieved. Balance can be achieved within a single workout, over two different exercise sessions or even across the space of a full week. This is done by evenly training muscle groups or by evenly training movement patterns. If a whole-body workout is devised, which may be suitable for a novice exerciser, it would be important that all movements or muscles were trained evenly within a single workout. Examples of balancing out a workout are ensuring you include a balanced amount of pushing and pulling exercises or that the chest is trained evenly with the latissimus dorsi and trapezius muscles. Other body parts or movements would need to be treated similarly in a whole body workout.

As your ability improves it may be necessary to increase the work performed on each body part or movement pattern which can increase the length of a single workout too much. This is usually when a training programme progresses to balance the body over two different exercise sessions or across a whole week. For example in a three-day-a-week workout the emphasis could vary so that day one is pushing and a small amount of core exercises, day two is pulling and squatting and day three is lunging and a different range of core exercises. While core training is performed on two different days the volume of work on each day would be half as much so that the two days combined would balance out with the other movement patterns. The recovery period between the third workout of the week and the first workout of the following week would be two days long so as to ensure adequate regeneration for the core muscles between workouts. Recovery between the other workouts would only be one day as different body parts are being trained so this will be sufficient each time.

CORE TRAINING

Core training refers to using the muscles in the mid-section of the body as the primary muscles responsible for performing the required movements for an exercise. In suspended fitness training the muscles that surround the torso and control movement between the pelvis and the ribs are involved to some degree in stabilising the body in almost all exercises. The concept of specifically training the core muscles during suspension training may therefore seem a little unnecessary. In most suspended exercises the core muscles are largely helping to stabilise the body so that other

target muscles can be worked more effectively. It is exactly this reason why the targeted core muscles and movements should be left until the end of a workout. If the core muscles are targeted earlier in a workout and become fatigued, this may compromise the quality of technique in other exercises that follow where the core is needed to help stabilise and control unwanted movements.

If we go back to the earlier example of seven exercises that were selected for an advanced exerciser new to suspended fitness training and apply the exercise order guidelines then one way these could be addressed is as follows:

1. Hanging ice skater (challenge 7 – see page 98)
2. Jumping sprint starts (challenge 6 – see page 102)
3. Hip thrust narrow row and reach (challenge 5 – see page 78)
4. Low to high straight-arm pull (challenge 5 – see page 75)
5. Single-leg squats (challenge 4 – see page 41)
6. Suspended squat jumps (challenge 4 – see page 42)
7. Suspended plank with rotational reach (challenge 5 – see page 110)

As all the selected exercises in the list involve large muscle groups then the exercises are weighed up and ordered in relation to their level of technical complexity with the specific core exercise left to the end. This is not the only way in which these exercises can be ordered, but it does offer a workable solution. The programme would still work fairly effectively even if exercises 1 and 2 were switched around. Exercises 3 and 4 or exercises 5 and 6 could also be switched and the programme would still function well enough.

Once all the exercises have been selected and a draft order created it is always good practice to double check that each of the exercise order rules has not been compromised.

SETS, REPS AND REST

The next stage is to apply a suitable set and repetition scheme to the exercises that have been selected and ordered. Each set needs to be balanced out with an appropriate rest period to allow for acute fatigue to dissipate and for muscles to replenish ready for the next set. The following guidelines offer some direction in relation to the training objective and suitable rest.

WARM-UP AND COOL-DOWN

Once the main component of an exercise session has been determined then an appropriate warm-up and cool-down can be planned to meet the needs of the intended session. A warm-up should consist of a brief cardiovascular pulse-raising activity and some dynamic mobility work targeted

to prepare and activate the body parts and movements to be used within the main session workout. The cardiovascular activity need only last between 3–5 minutes in most cases to raise heart rate and increase muscle temperature sufficiently. The key is to begin at a slower and lighter intensity and gradually increase to a moderate pace and intensity during the few short minutes of cardiovascular activity. The application of aerobic exercise such as a run on a treadmill or elliptical trainer, a cycle on a stationary bike, or a few minutes on a rower will normally deliver the required effect. At home some jogging on the spot, jumping jacks, skipping or burpees would help provide the same effect. Dynamic activities to improve range of motion and muscle activation can be selected from the range of mobilisation exercises outlined previously in chapter 5. The key consideration is that the mobility work selected is based around similar movements that are scheduled to follow in the main exercise component of the workout.

Table 8.1	Typical set and repetition scheme			
Objective	Reps	Sets per exercise	Rest period (seconds) between sets	Load
Joint stabilisation or rehabilitation	4–15 (depending on joint function)	1–2	60–120	light
Muscular endurance and/or tone	13–20	1–3	30–60	light to moderate
Body-weight strength	6–12	2–5	45–90	moderate to heavy
Speed power	6–12	2–4	90–180	moderate

A cool-down should be included immediately after the main exercise session to assist in returning to a normal resting state. This typically consists of a gradual pulse-lowering activity and some appropriate stretching to restore muscle length or further develop flexibility. Whether or not a cardiovascular activity is required to help cool the body down is dependent on the intensity of the final exercise. If a high-intensity exercise was used to finish the main session then it would be appropriate to apply 2–3 minutes of cardiovascular activity that starts at a moderate level and gradually lower intensity to finish at a light level of activity. For example, a gentle jog reducing to a brisk walk then a slow walk would suffice. Static stretching activities can be selected from the range offered previously in chapter 8.

Generally the main workout will help to dictate the body parts and muscles that need stretching. Refer to the primary muscle groups used in each of the exercises and plan to apply an appropriate static stretch for each one. Also if an individual has any chronically tight muscles then these should also be stretched even if they were not worked as part of the training session. Chronically tight muscles would benefit from several developmental phases of static stretching to help increase their length and lower muscular tension.

BEGINNER LEVEL PROGRAMMING

If you have not exercised in a while or suspended fitness training is new to you then there are a number of considerations to take into account when devising a training programme. Weighing each of these factors in the balance and determining how they should influence your training programme will likely play a role in the success of the resulting exercise plan. Beginners will more likely:

- Struggle with new exercise techniques
- Have decreased ability to fully activate muscle tissue
- Have reduced muscle tissue tolerance
- Require longer recovery times

These factors will mean that you will need to choose exercises that have easy-to-grasp technical requirements and that will allow for lower levels of intensity performance. Jumping or other similar powerful exercises are too intense for most beginner exercisers. Setting the acute variables such as sets, repetitions and rest periods also requires judgement to provide a sufficient stimulus to bring about adaptation, but not so much that the individual cannot complete the workout or ends up suffering from too much post-exercise muscle soreness. A single exercise per body part, endurance repetition range, two sets per exercise and short rest periods are usually sufficient stimulus for a beginner. The exercise challenge ratings for beginner exercisers should generally range from 1 to 3. The following workout plan provides an example of a whole body workout suitable for somebody who is relatively new to exercise and has not used suspended fitness training previously.

INTERMEDIATE LEVEL PROGRAMMING

An intermediate exercise plan would be appropriate for an individual who has been regularly using suspended fitness training as part of their training programme for 6 to 12 weeks. The introduction

WARM UP				
Exercise	Speed/rpm	Incline/Level	Duration	Notes
CV: Cross trainer	80-120 rpm	3-6	5 mins	Gradual increase in intensity from level 3 at 80rpm up to level 6 at 120rpm

Dynamic mobility: 8-10 reps for each mobilisation – hamstrings, quadriceps, calf complex, iliopsoas, gluteals, latissimus dorsi, abdominals, pectorals

MAIN SESSION				TRAINING RECORD				
Exercise	Sets/reps	Rest	Notes	Date:	Date:	Date:	Date:	Date:
Suspended squats	2 × 15	30-60 sec	This programme plan has 2 execution options:					
Suspended side lunge	2 × 15	30-60 sec						
Chest press	2 × 15	30-60 sec	Perform 2 sets of each exercise in order					
Narrow grip hanging row	2 × 15	30-60 sec						
Reverse flye	2 × 15	30-60 sec	Perform a single set of all 8 exercises without any rest in circuit fashion then repeat a second time after 2-3 minutes recovery					
Hanging biceps curl	2 × 15	30-60 sec						
Overhead triceps press	2 × 15	30-60 sec						
Suspended plank	2 × 30-45 sec	30-60 sec						

COOL DOWN				
Exercise	Speed/rpm	Incline/Level	Duration	Notes
CV: Treadmill	9–4 mph	0%	3 mins	Gradual reduction in intensity

Static stretches: 20-30 seconds hold for each stretch – quadriceps, hamstrings, gluteals, calf complex, pectorals, latissimus dorsi, biceps, triceps, abdominals

Figure 8.2 Beginner programme A1

of a more challenging training regime would be dependent upon successful progress and improvement during the previous stages of training and not just simply reaching the six-week mark.

There are numerous ways in which a programme can be changed to progress onwards, including:

• Selecting new exercises

WARM UP				
Exercise	Speed/ rpm	Incline /Level	Duration	Notes
CV: Treadmill	4 – 10 mph	0%	5 mins	Gradual increase in intensity from level brisk walk at 4mph up to running at 10mph

Dynamic mobility: 8-10 reps each mobilisation – hamstrings, quadriceps, calf complex, iliopsoas, gluteals, latissimus dorsi, abdominals, pectorals

MAIN SESSION				TRAINING RECORD				
Exercise	Sets/ reps	Rest	Notes	Date:	Date:	Date:	Date:	Date:
Single leg squat	3 × 10 L&R	90 sec	Keep slow and controlled - perform left and right sides before rest is earned					
Squat jump start	2 × 12	90 sec						
Chest press	2 × 10	90 sec	Perform one set of each exercise non-stop before the 90 second rest					
Chest flye	2 × 10							
Single grip narrow row and reach	3 × 10 L&R	90 sec	Increase angle of load – perform left and right sides before rest is earned					
Reverse flye	2 × 12	60 sec	Increased angle of load					
Inverted press	2 × 10	60 sec						
Hanging biceps curl	2 × 12	60 sec	Increased angle of load					
Suspended jackknife	3 × 15	60 sec	Keep repetition speed slow and controlled					

COOL DOWN				
Exercise	Speed/ rpm	Incline /Level	Duration	Notes
CV: Stationary bicycle	80–50	6–3	3 mins	Gradual reduction in intensity and pedal speed

Static stretches: 20-30 seconds hold for each stretch – quadriceps, hamstrings, gluteals, calf complex, pectorals, latissimus dorsi, biceps, deltoids, hip flexors, abdominals

Figure 8.3 Intermediate programme B1

WARM UP				
Exercise	Speed/ rpm	Incline / Level	Duration	Notes
CV: Treadmill	4 – 10 mph	0%	5 mins	Gradual increase in intensity from level brisk walk at 4mph up to running at 10mph

Dynamic mobility: 8-10 reps each mobilisation – hamstrings, quadriceps, calf complex, iliopsoas, gluteals, latissimus dorsi, abdominals, pectorals

MAIN SESSION				TRAINING RECORD				
Exercise	Sets/ reps	Rest	Notes	Date:	Date:	Date:	Date:	Date:
Suspended squat jump	3 x 15	90 sec						
Suspended lunge with multi-directional reach	2 x 12 R&L	90 sec	Perform one set each side before earning rest – with 6 directions of reach the full cycle will be completed twice in 12 reps					
Alternating wide chest press	3 x 12	90 sec	Perform one set of each exercise non-stop before earning a rest					
Low to high straight arm pull	3 x 12							
Hip thrust to row	2 x 15	60 sec						
Suspended walking plank	2 x 8 reps	60 sec						
Suspended cycling jack knife	2 x 20	60 sec						

COOL DOWN				
Exercise	Speed/ rpm	Incline / Level	Duration	Notes
CV: Stationary bicycle	80 - 50	6 - 3	3 mins	Gradual reduction in intensity and pedal speed

Static stretches: 20-30 seconds hold for each stretch – quadriceps, hamstrings, gluteals, calf complex, pectorals, latissimus dorsi, biceps, deltoids, hip flexors, abdominals

Figure 8.4 Intermediate programme B2

- Changing target repetitions
- Increasing the number of sets
- Adjusting rest periods between sets
- Removing rest periods between exercises
- Increasing the angle of loading
- Increasing or decreasing repetition speed
- Increasing exercise complexity

Sometimes there is a temptation to progress too far too soon and to completely rework the whole training programme so that it looks nothing like the original programme that was used during the beginner stages. In most cases this rapid change of direction may be too much too soon. Usually it is good practice to keep some elements of an intermediate programme similar to the original beginner phase workouts. There is a balance that needs to be struck between progressing the exercise programme to sustain fitness development and retaining some familiarity so that the individual feels capable of meeting the demands of the revised workout. After working hard for 6 to 12 weeks to master a beginner programme it can be demotivating to feel like the updated programme has returned the exerciser to step one. This is why some exercises should still be within the familiar challenge rating of 2 or 3, as in a beginner programme. Other exercises selected to be part of an intermediate programme should progress up to as high as 5 on the challenge rating. The exercises that remain at the lower challenge rating will still need to progress in terms of sets, repetitions and rest.

The other circumstance where an intermediate programme may be a suitable option is when an experienced exerciser who has a good foundation of fitness training begins using suspended fitness training for the first time. While they may already have good physical attributes that will serve them well, their lack of familiarity with suspended training justifies that they do not start at an advanced level while they learn new exercise techniques and develop the needed movement control. They are not a fitness beginner, just a beginner to this specific form of training, hence the compromise of starting at an intermediate level. A training programme for this type of individual will still need to address the overall training objective and current physical abilities. It would be useful to allow a workout that covers the whole body so that they develop good all-round exercise technique. The exercise challenge rating for this type of client would best be selected from exercises in the range of 3–5.

ADVANCED PROGRAMME DESIGN

Once an individual masters a range of intermediate exercise techniques and adapts to the training intensity and exercise challenge, it is time to progress onwards to a more advanced training programme. It is recommended that an individual, who started as a beginner, have between 16 to 24 weeks of progressive suspended fitness training by the time they progress to an advanced programme.

When creating more advanced training programmes there are many options available to manipulate the variables and increase the challenge, including:

- designing split routines
- progressing the training phase
- manipulating work to rest ratios
- applying advanced training systems

- combining with other training modalities
- increasing the movement complexity

The use of split routines becomes very helpful as training capacity increases. If a whole body workout continues to be used the set, repetitions and number of exercises generally progresses to a point where the volume of exercise and time it takes to complete becomes too high. Therefore to reduce the time spent performing each workout, and to ensure progression continues, the body or movement patterns can be split up across different days, for example:

- Day 1: Push, squat and core
- Day 2: Pull, lunge and core

It may also be important to switch to a different training phase. Instead of working in an endurance or body-weight strength range, it may be helpful to progress some exercises up into a power phase. The different exercises can also have some suspension-friendly advanced-training systems applied such as supersets, tri sets or a PHA circuit. Each of these systems help to increase the training density and to boost the stimulus to bring increased gains, providing recovery between workouts continues to be effective. It would be useful to quickly define what each of these advanced training systems entails.

- **Supersets** – require that two exercises are performed back to back without any rest to comprise a single set. These exercises should either be for the same muscle group or movement pattern or they can also be opposing muscle groups or movement patterns e.g., two push exercises together or alternatively a push and a pull exercise pair.

- **Tri sets** – are much the same as supersets except that there are three exercises that make up the non-stop training set. Tri sets are normally three exercises focused on the same muscle group or movement pattern performed back to back.
- **PHA circuit** – PHA stands for peripheral heart action. In simple terms this is combining a group of three exercises together with a short aerobic training component. The three resistance exercises focus on three different body parts that require the shunting of blood from one area to another during the circuit. The most common type of PHA circuit will usually include one push, one pull and one legs exercise with an aerobic exercise at the end. A rest is only allowed after one set of all four exercises has been performed and then the circuit may be repeated again.

Each of these training systems effectively increases the exercise density as it squeezes more exercises into less time by removing rest periods. These training systems tend to be very intense and increase the metabolic demand on the body with greater fatigue and more lactic acid build up in the targeted muscles. Lactic acid is a by-product of high energy output in the muscles and is associated with an intense burning sensation in the muscles that decreases performance. Therefore a word of caution with regard to the three advanced training systems: they should not be over-used. One or two selected methods in a single workout are more than enough. The training programme that follows provides two advanced workouts that form part of the same training week that would be performed twice each week in a four-day training week.

WARM UP				
Exercise	Speed/ rpm	Incline / Level	Duration	Notes
CV: Rower	25-30 spm	7	5 mins	Gradually increase intensity from 2:20 min/ 500m to 1:50 min/500m

Dynamic mobility: 8-10 reps each mobilisation – hamstrings, quadriceps, calf complex, iliopsoas, gluteals, pectorals, abdominals

MAIN SESSION				TRAINING RECORD				
Exercise	Sets / reps	Rest	Notes	Date:	Date:	Date:	Date:	Date:
High and wide chest flye	3 × 8 R&L	PHA circuit: 4 exercises non-stop then 120 sec rest	Flye right and left for each repetition					
Transverse squat jumps	3 × 8		Jump right and left for each repetition					
Suspended plank with rotational reach	3 × 8		Reach right and left for each repetition					
Treadmill	3 × 1 min		Run at 70% intensity (9-12mph)					
Squat jump start	2 × 10	90 sec	Perform both sets non-stop as a superset to earn rest					
Single leg squat jump	2 × 10							
Walking suspended press up	3 × 12	90 sec						
Reverse cycling plank	3 × 12	90 sec						

COOL DOWN				
Exercise	Speed/ rpm	Incline / Level	Duration	Notes
CV: Bike	80 – 50 rpm	6 – 3	3 mins	Gradual reduction in speed and intensity evenly across time

Static stretches: 20-30 seconds hold for each stretch – quadriceps, hamstrings, gluteals, calf complex, hip flexors, pectorals, triceps, abdominals, erector spinae

Figure 8.5 Advanced programme C1

WARM UP				
Exercise	Speed/ rpm	Incline / Level	Duration	Notes
CV: Cross trainer	100-150 rpm	4-8	5 mins	Gradual increase in intensity from level 4 at 100 rpm up to level 8 at 150 rpm

Dynamic mobility: 8-10 reps each mobilisation – hamstrings, quadriceps, calf complex, iliopsoas, gluteals, latissimus dorsi, biceps, abdominals

MAIN SESSION				TRAINING RECORD				
Exercise	Sets / reps	Rest	Notes	Date:	Date:	Date:	Date:	Date:
Hip thrust to row	3 x 15	Tri-set: 3 sets nonstop then 120 sec rest	Powerful positive contraction with controlled return to start					
Wide hanging row	3 x 12		Maintain a steady, controlled pace					
Single arm wide row with single leg squat	3 x 10		Only half squat depth required					
Suspended lunge with multi-directional reach	3 x 12	90 sec						
Hanging ice skater	3 x 12	90 sec						
Suspended body saw	3 x 10	90 sec	Superset both exercises non-stop before earning rest					
Suspended walking jack knife	3 x 10							

COOL DOWN				
Exercise	Speed/ rpm	Incline / Level	Duration	Notes
CV: Treadmill	9 - 4 mph	0%	3 mins	Gradual reduction in intensity

Static stretches: 20-30 seconds hold for each stretch – quadriceps, hamstrings, gluteals, calf complex, iliopsoas, adductors, latissimus dorsi, biceps, posterior deltoids, abdominals

Figure 8.6 Advanced programme C2

These exercise programmes show examples of how different exercises can be varied to form effective training sessions for different ability levels, to keep workouts creative and exciting. There are many ways in which groups of exercises can be combined to deliver creative and exciting workouts. The intention in this chapter has been to help teach the basic principles for developing and planning your own training programmes. Understanding and applying the principles of programme design is much more powerful than simply following a range of previously designed workouts without any understanding as to why they have been put together in the way that they have. Too often it is the fear of making mistakes that stop individuals from moving forward in their physical fitness goals. Be positive and experiment with new ideas that meet and guide you towards your physical training objectives. Follow these five simple steps to successful programming and you will enjoy designing and applying your fitness training for months to come.

1. Select a range of exercises that are goal oriented
2. Determine the exercise order for the workout by following the four basic exercise ordering rules
3. Plan in sets, repetitions and rest that meet individual ability and training phase objectives
4. Design a brief warm-up and cool-down to prepare for and stretch out the muscles involved in the workout
5. Adjust and progress the workout regularly to prevent training from going stale and to move little by little towards short, medium and long term goals

Remember that regular change and progression are an essential part of seeing success with a suspended fitness training programme!

KEPT IN SUSPENSE 9

One of the greatest challenges to even the most committed exerciser is long-term adherence to a training programme. Often individuals are found applying exercise in a very cyclic or seasonal pattern, full of drive and enthusiasm during certain periods of the year and then struggling for motivation later on. The New Year surge in gym attendance and exercise uptake is a good example of this cyclic pattern. The change to a new season, especially spring time, often inspires people to become more active and get fitter.

Another common pattern is to work really hard on a new training programme for a few weeks; just enough to see a little progress before running out of steam a little too soon. This is often followed by a period where exercise ceases completely for a month or two only then to pick it up again later and simply repeat the same process.

Many people may also be familiar with the weekend warrior who regularly trains hard on Saturdays and Sundays but is nowhere to be seen during the rest of the week.

These boom-and-bust training approaches, whether a weekly cycle or over longer periods of time, tend to lead to little more than fitness maintenance at best. It is rare that such extreme cyclical training, an all-or-nothing approach, will lead

to real progress and fitness development. Rather than swing from 100 per cent commitment to no commitment at all it is better to apply a less vigorous, but more sustainable approach to exercise. Integrating an appropriate exercise pattern into life that can become a regular, enjoyable habit is simply a better solution to achieving long-term success.

Part of the challenge in creating exercise habits that fit in with life is the fact that most individuals try to fit in with the typical, modern cultural practices around exercise. For example, training three times per week on Monday, Wednesday and Fridays, at least one hour per exercise session and even dividing a workout into aerobic and resistance training components are all commonly practised beliefs around exercise. Without ever placing an expectation on any of my clients over the many years that I have worked in the fitness industry, the large majority would state that they wanted to attend three times per week for an hour at a time. This is interesting considering the national UK average for gym attendance is closer to twice per week. Training three times per week for an hour may be too little to sustain physical progress for one person, while for another it may be too much to fit in with their on-going life commitments and therefore destined to fail from the outset. The individual with a busy life will usually struggle to fit exercise into their regular schedule. Children, relationships, employment, home improvements and social commitments simply are higher up on their priority scale and value hierarchy. Trying to fit the standard norms and beliefs regarding exercise to their already fast-paced and sometimes chaotic life will usually not work, certainly not in the long term. It would seem appropriate to break the norm right from the outset and apply a different set of guidelines that have a better chance of fitting in with modern lifestyles. Some potential exercise options could include:

- 30 minutes training, 4 times per week
- 1 hour training, 2 times per week, evenly split over the week
- 20 minutes training, 5 times per week
- 45 minutes training, twice at the weekend, once mid-week
- 2 x 30-minute morning sessions, 1 x 1 hour evening session spread out across the week

These are by no means the only other options available, but they are included to show that a different approach can be taken to training frequency that will still have benefits and help create regular habits that can be sustained in the long-term. Indeed, an individual may find that they need to switch their attendance workout habits from week to week depending on their other commitments in life. This adaptable approach to physical exercise can help prevent a boom-or-bust cycle of training. It prevents a missed training session here or there negatively impacting upon motivation and leading to a collapse in sticking to an exercise programme.

It is natural to prefer predictable routines. Many people go through the same daily habits and processes during their day without fully being consciously aware of it. Routine can help us feel safe, secure and normal. When introducing something new, like an exercise programme, this can initially upset the routine and it can feel like an effort partly because it is outside of the routine we have created for ourselves. One of the ways in which an exercise programme can feel routine even sooner is to stick with the exact same programme so that even the actual workout becomes a familiar routine itself. After a few weeks of faithfully working through an exercise plan, the challenge of the programme is soon within our physical ability as the body adapts to the stimulus. Once this physical compensation has happened and the body is comfortable with the exercise that has been programmed that a change is needed. The problem is that this also tends to be the time when we begin to feel that the exercise itself has become a normal part of our routine. Now that exercise feels routine it is common to find a reluctance to shake things up and change the workout. After working so hard to make the exercise programme feel routine and part of our habits and regular cycles it can seem unsettling to change things and then have a new routine to have to adapt to again. However, this is exactly what needs to happen. Regular change with regard to exercise programming is an important element of your on-going success.

Introducing new elements to your training programme is vital for interest and motivation. The problem with routines is that they soon become mundane and lack the drive or motivation needed to maintain interest and enjoyment. Routine may keep you going for a while, but in relation to exercise a lack of interest and motivation soon becomes a bigger factor and when boredom sets in failure to adhere to exercise soon becomes the result. Right from the outset of an exercise programme the expectation and objective should be to progress to the next point where the exercises will change and need upgrading. We live in a world where getting an upgrade is seen to be very desirable, for example the latest mobile phone or software upgrade. This is the attitude we need to have with regard to our exercise programme. The reward to mastering the previous programme and experiencing the benefits it had to offer is to get an exercise programme upgrade! We need to seek these changes in our training routine. This will help to keep interest and motivation high and it will help to ensure that your body is still being challenged and the physical stimulus is sufficient to require growth and adaptation. Therefore, the one aspect regarding your training that must become routine is a healthy expectation and need for regular updates and adjustments to your exercise programme.

Once you have worked out an exercise programme that is right for you, and have thought about ways to incorporate your new training regime into your day-to-day life, you will come to see that suspended fitness training – whether by itself or in conjunction with other training programmes – is an enjoyable way of achieving your fitness objectives. Invest in a training system and you can take your fitness programme anywhere, which may be particularly desirable if you have a busy lifestyle.

Above all I hope this book has given you the tools to feel confident in undertaking suspended fitness training and that you quickly see results, reach your fitness objectives and, most of all, have fun. Happy suspending!

Quick Suspended Exercise Index

GLOSSARY

Abduction: movement in the frontal plane away from the midline of the body

Adduction: movement in the frontal plane towards the midline of the body

Angle of loading: the angle of the body in relation to the ground when performing a suspended fitness exercise

Biomechanics: the study of the mechanics of the body, particularly the forces exerted by muscles and gravity on the skeletal structure

Carabiner: a metal coupling link with a safety closure

Centre of gravity: the place in the body where weight is evenly dispersed and all parts are in balance

Co-contraction: when muscles on both sides of a joint engage and pull to hold the joint motionless or to help stabilise a joint more effectively during movement

Compound exercise: an exercise that utilises more than one joint as part of the primary mechanism

Contraindication: a condition or factor that serves as a reason not to apply a treatment (in this case exercise) due to an increased risk of harm

Dynamic mobility: using rhythmical joint motion to help lengthen muscle tissue and improve joint mechanics, fluidity and range of movement

Effort arm: the distance between the pivot point and the site where effort or force is applied

Endurance training: training devised to improve muscular ability to repeatedly contract without undue fatigue; usually higher repetitions, lighter loads, low volume sets and shorter rest periods

Exercise complexity: the degree of technical difficulty in performing an exercise

Extension: the bending of a joint so that the angle between the bones increases

Flexion: the bending of a joint so that the angle between the bones decreases

Frontal plane movement: side to side movement towards and away from the midline of the body e.g. abduction and adduction

Hypertrophy training: training devised to increase muscular size by increasing the cross sectional area of muscle fibres; usually medium repetitions, moderate loads, high volume sets and short to medium rest

Isolation exercise: an exercise that utilises only one joint as part of the primary mechanism

Lateral: towards the sides or away from the middle

Mechanical advantage: the force amplification achieved by using a tool, mechanical device or machine system

Medial: towards the middle or away from the sides

Moment arm: the length between a joint and the line of force acting upon that joint

Momentum: the strength or force that something has when it is moving, dependent upon its total mass and velocity

Muscle spindle: sensory receptors found deep within the muscle tissue that respond to changes in muscle length and the rate of length change

Pendulum effect: the regular, swinging motion of a pendulum by the action of gravity and acquired momentum; the influence of gravity upon an object that swings beneath a pivot point

Pivot point: the central turning point of a rotational system

Proprioception: the unconscious perception of movement and spatial orientation arising from sensory receptors within the body itself

Resistance arm: the distance between the pivot point or axis and the point where resistance to force is applied

Sagittal plane movement: forwards or backwards movement away from the midline of the body e.g. flexion and extension

Spinal alignment: holding the spine in position where each vertebrae is evenly loaded one on top of the other to form a natural 'S' shaped curve

Static stretching: holding muscle tissue in an elongated position without movement in an effort to either increase or restore muscle length

Stretch reflex: a nervous reflex where lengthening a muscle causes a stimulus to contract and shorten the same muscle

Torque: the measure of the turning force of an object around a pivot point

Transverse plane movement: rotational movement around the longitudinal axis of the body e.g. medial or lateral rotation

Webbing: strong, closely woven fabric used for making items such as straps and belts

INDEX

Page numbers in *italic* refer to illustrations